Immunopathology of Chronic Respiratory Diseases

Edited by Seyyed Shamsadin Athari and Entezar Mehrabi Nasab

Published in London, United Kingdom

Immunopathology of Chronic Respiratory Diseases
http://dx.doi.org/10.5772/intechopen.1004671
Edited by Seyyed Shamsadin Athari and Entezar Mehrabi Nasab

Contributors
Alka Singh, Ayesha Fiaz, Irum Shahzad, Kiran Dobhal, Lucia Vietri, Maria Daniela Mot, Marian Gabriel, Oyindamola Akinso, Paula Irina Barata, Qurat Ul Ain, Ruchika Garg, Terry Chin, Tugba Raika Kıran, Wajida Perveen, Yasha Sajjad

First published in London, United Kingdom, 2025 by IntechOpen
IntechOpen is the global imprint of INTECHOPEN LIMITED, registered in England and Wales, registration number: 11086078, 167-169 Great Portland Street, London, W1W 5PF, United Kingdom

For EU product safety concerns: IN TECH d.o.o., Prolaz Marije Krucifikse Kozulić 3, 51000 Rijeka, Croatia, info@intechopen.com or visit our website at intechopen.com.

British Library Cataloguing-in-Publication Data
A catalogue record for this book is available from the British Library

Immunopathology of Chronic Respiratory Diseases
Edited by Seyyed Shamsadin Athari and Entezar Mehrabi Nasab
p. cm.
Print ISBN 978-1-83634-296-0
Online ISBN 978-1-83634-295-3
eBook (PDF) ISBN 978-1-83634-297-7

Meet the editors

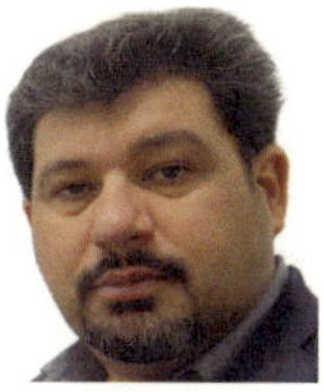

Dr. Seyyed Shamsadin Athari is an assistant professor of immunology in the Department of Immunology, School of Medicine, Zanjan University of Medical Sciences, Zanjan, Iran, and has an allergy and asthma toxicology postdoctorate and an asthma management and controlling network fellowship. He has published over 250 manuscripts in international journals in immunology, allergy, and asthma and has written over 35 books. He is also on the editorial board of more than 90 international journals in medical sciences, has inventions in medical sciences, and has recorded gene sequences in a gene bank. Dr. Athari has been invited as a top speaker to more than 50 international congresses and symposiums and has received scientific awards from different scientific societies as a young top researcher and young scientist.

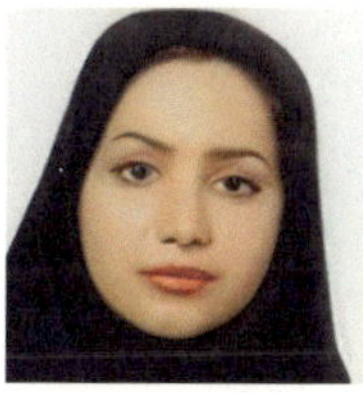

Dr. Entezar Mehrabi Nasab, MD, is a cardiologist specializing in cardiovascular diseases and holds a fellowship in interventional clinical electrophysiology. She completed her residency and fellowship at the Tehran Heart Center, Tehran University of Medical Sciences, Iran. She has published more than 40 scientific articles in international journals. She has been an invited speaker at more than 30 international congresses. Dr. Mehrabi Nasab has received awards from different scientific societies.

Contents

Preface

The role of immunity in the pathogenesis of various pulmonary diseases, particularly interstitial lung diseases, is receiving increasing attention as mechanistic discoveries advance our knowledge in this field. Immune-mediated pulmonary diseases exhibit clinical and immunological heterogeneity. They can be classified etiologically into connective tissue-related, exposure-related, idiopathic, and other miscellaneous pulmonary diseases, including sarcoidosis and posttransplant interstitial lung diseases. Immunological diseases of the lung include a diverse group of disorders characterized by activation of the innate and adaptive arms of the immune system. In some cases, the immune response is localized to the lung, such as in idiopathic pulmonary fibrosis and cryptogenic organizing pneumonia, whereas in connective tissue diseases, the lung is one of the affected organs. As a result, the respiratory tract is exposed to inhaled particles, and the defense mechanisms clear most particles from the upper airway. The immune pathogenesis of many diseases is not well defined and likely involves immune system dysfunction, abnormal healing, chronic inflammation, or a combination of these, often in the context of genetic predisposition. The respiratory tract deserves special attention in the discussion of immunity. Because of its gas exchange function, the respiratory tract is a stage for a constant conflict between the immune system and external exposures that enter the airways with each breath.

Therefore, in the current book, an effort has been made to introduce and present new aspects of the immunopathology of chronic respiratory diseases and the role of immune responses in both their pathogenesis and protection. We hope this book offers a new perspective on the control and treatment of chronic respiratory diseases.

Seyyed Shamsadin Athari
Zanjan University of Medical Sciences,
Zanjan, Iran

Entezar Mehrabi Nasab
Tehran University of Medical Sciences,
Teheran, Iran

Chapter 1

Global Childhood Asthma: Caregivers Knowledge, Attitude and Management Practices

Oyindamola Akinso

Abstract

This chapter examines childhood asthma, a widespread chronic condition affecting millions of children worldwide. It focuses on the current understanding, attitudes, and management practices surrounding this condition. The chapter begins by emphasizing the critical role of caregivers' knowledge and attitudes in managing their children's asthma. A lack of awareness about common asthma triggers among many caregivers often leads to suboptimal control of the condition. Challenges in diagnosing and managing childhood asthma in economically disadvantaged areas are also discussed, including limited access to healthcare services, shortages of trained professionals, and inadequate diagnostic tools. These obstacles frequently contribute to delayed diagnoses and ineffective management strategies. The chapter underscores the importance of targeted educational interventions to improve caregivers' understanding and responses to asthma triggers. By equipping caregivers with the necessary knowledge and resources, prevention strategies aim to enhance asthma outcomes, ultimately improving the quality of life for children in low-resource settings. Case studies and real-world examples illustrate effective approaches and common challenges in managing childhood asthma. The goal is to provide a comprehensive resource that deepens understanding and contributes to better global outcomes for children living with asthma.

Keywords: asthma management behavior, pediatric asthma, childhood asthma management, global health, caregivers, wheezing, asthma triggers, rural communities, asthma risk factors, and global burden of asthma

1. Introduction

Asthma is one of the most common chronic inflammatory diseases that are associated with a reversible narrowing and obstruction of the airways and clinical manifestations such as recurrent episodes of wheezing, coughing, chest tightness, and breathing difficulties [1, 2]. Asthma is not just a public health problem, but a global health issue. Globally, asthma is known to be one of the leading causes of respiratory disorder; with more than 235 million people affected with the disease worldwide; and a global prevalence ranging from 1–18% [3, 4]. Global asthma prevalence has drastically increased worldwide, particularly in low and middle-income countries.

According to the World Health Organization (WHO), approximately 235 million people are currently suffering from asthma; and the disease is often common among children [4]. Asthma is a global health problem, not just an epidemic in high-income countries but also a huge public health problem in all other countries regardless of their level of development. According to the latest reports from WHO, the highest prevalence of asthma-related deaths occurs in low and lower-middle-income countries [4].

At the same time, studies have shown a significant rise in the prevalence of childhood asthma in developing countries compared to developed nations [5]. Evidence from these studies highlights that the highest burden of childhood asthma is found in low- and middle-income countries, particularly in regions such as Southeast Asia, Africa, the Western Pacific, and the Eastern Mediterranean [6, 7]. While these reports demonstrate a wide variation in asthma prevalence across different countries [8], the International Study of Asthma and Allergies in Childhood (ISAAC) Phase 1 showed that asthma symptom prevalence ranged from less than 5% in some developing countries to more than 20% in certain developed nations [8]. Despite the limited data available, the growing rates of childhood asthma in low-resource settings highlight an urgent need for a better understanding of caregivers' knowledge, attitudes, and management practices, which play a critical role in addressing the global burden of this condition.

The highest prevalence of asthma in developing countries is observed among children and young adults living in rural areas and resource-poor settings, where healthcare providers are scarce and educational information for caregivers is often lacking [2, 6]. For instance, in rural Nigeria, the factors that contribute to the rising incidence of asthma among children aged 1–5 years remain poorly understood [7]. Evidence from previous research indicates that inadequate asthma management and control practices by parents and caregivers are key factors behind the increase in asthma episodes among children, particularly those living in low-resource communities [9]. The consequences of childhood asthma extend beyond school absenteeism, hospitalizations, and emergency room visits; the burden on caregivers, who are primarily responsible for managing their children's asthma, significantly affects their physical and mental well-being.

As the prevalence of childhood asthma continues to rise globally, many studies have shifted their focus to identifying the risk factors associated with asthma and finding effective ways to prevent recurrent asthma episodes in both children and adults. However, few studies have examined the direct impact of caregiver knowledge, attitudes, and practices on asthma management in young children. Understanding these aspects is crucial, as improved caregiver education and support could play a critical role in reducing asthma-related morbidity and enhancing the quality of life for both children and their families.

2. Caregivers of asthmatic children in poor resource settings

In many developing countries, particularly in settings with limited resources, there is still a lack of comprehensive understanding regarding caregivers' experiences with childhood asthma and their management practices. In countries like Nigeria, research on caregivers' knowledge and approaches to managing childhood asthma remains scarce [7]. Some studies have shown that parents of children with asthma may hold poor knowledge or misconceptions about the disease and its treatment [9, 10]. Common misconceptions include beliefs that asthma can be cured, that it is contagious, or that traditional treatments or homemade remedies are more effective than modern medicine. Additionally, many caregivers mistakenly believe that inhalers are addictive or ineffective and that asthma necessarily limits a child's ability to exercise [9, 10]. These beliefs contribute to significant gaps in knowledge about the disease's symptoms, diagnosis, and appropriate management [11]. Without accurate knowledge of asthma, caregivers may fail to recognize the early warning signs or respond appropriately, which can lead to worsening symptoms and poor health outcomes for the child [9].

One of the significant challenges in managing asthma in children under the age of five is the difficulty in diagnosing the condition at such a young age. Since children in this age group cannot easily articulate their symptoms, healthcare providers rely heavily on caregivers to describe what they have observed. The ability of caregivers to accurately report symptoms such as coughing or wheezing is critical, yet these symptoms can often indicate other respiratory conditions rather than asthma [12]. Consequently, delays in diagnosis can occur, preventing the child from receiving timely and appropriate care. According to the American Academy of Allergy, Asthma, & Immunology (AAAI), although asthma is not curable, it can be managed effectively to prevent severe symptoms and complications [13].

Studies have indicated that if asthma symptoms are not controlled in childhood, they can persist in adulthood, becoming more severe and difficult to manage [2]. Proper management in early childhood is critical to reducing the risk of long-term morbidity and mortality associated with the disease [2]. However, managing asthma in children under the age of five is particularly challenging, as the treatment options available for older children may not be suitable for very young children and infants.

In developed countries like the United States, caregivers are provided with extensive support and information to help them manage their child's asthma effectively. A stepwise approach is often used, which focuses on minimizing asthma episodes through regular monitoring, avoiding triggers, and employing a combination of short-acting and long-term control medications. For instance, daily anti-inflammatory medications are prescribed to reduce airway inflammation, while short-acting drugs are used to treat symptoms during an asthma attack. Parents are also encouraged to keep detailed records of their child's symptoms and treatment response, enabling healthcare providers to develop and adjust an individualized asthma action plan. This proactive approach reduces suffering and hospital visits, ultimately lowering healthcare costs. Additionally, it has been shown to significantly decrease the frequency of asthma exacerbations and emergency department visits for children under five [12].

Unfortunately, these strategies have not been widely implemented in many developing countries. Caregivers in impoverished communities often face significant barriers to managing asthma effectively. Financial hardship, limited access to healthcare providers, and poor health infrastructure contribute to high asthma morbidity and mortality rates. Caregivers in these settings are often unable to afford or access the medications and treatments their children need [11]. Furthermore, the absence of adequate health education and support exacerbates the challenge, leaving many caregivers without the knowledge and resources to manage their child's asthma properly. Recently, Researchers collaborating on the CHILD Cohort Study (CHILD) have created a straightforward symptom-based screening tool designed to identify asthma risk in children as young as 2 years old. The Childhood Asthma Risk Tool (CHART) is designed for use by family doctors and nurses in low-resource primary care settings, as it is non-invasive, cost-free, and requires no special equipment. CHART tool

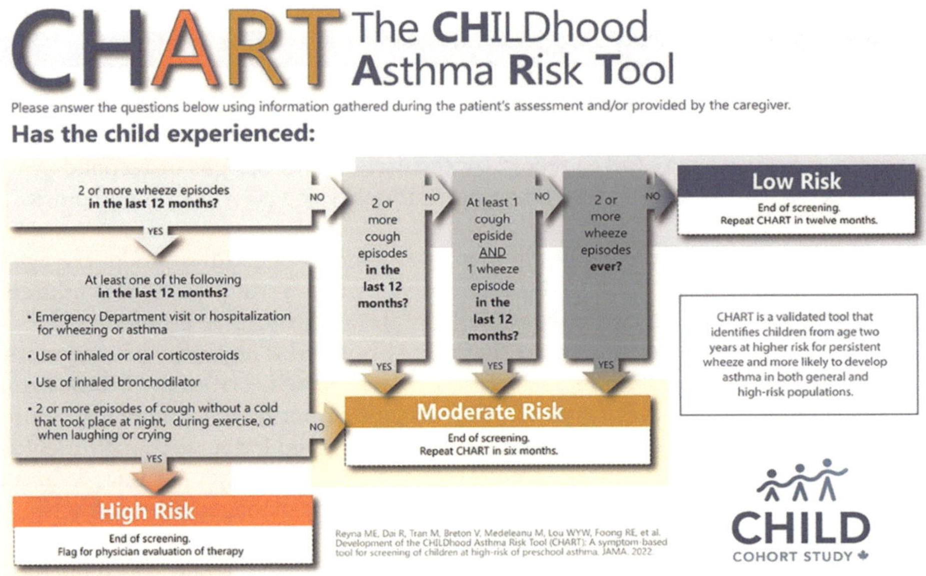

Figure 1.
CHART: The childhood asthma risk tool: The Childhood Asthma Risk Tool (CHART) is a symptom-based screening tool designed to identify young children at high risk of developing asthma Source: *Ref. [14]. Creative Commons Attribution (CC-BY) License. This figure is used under the Creative Commons Attribution (CC-BY) license.*

innovation facilitates earlier detection of asthma in children, allowing doctors to initiate treatment sooner. CHART predicts asthma risk in children, allowing primary caregivers to assess the likelihood of future asthma and persistent symptoms before age three. It categorizes risk levels as 'high,' 'moderate,' or 'low' and provides recommended follow-up actions for each category (**Figure 1**).

Caregivers of children with asthma in poor-resource settings face significant challenges in managing childhood asthma. Effective asthma management strategies, like those used in developed countries, are urgently needed in these regions to reduce asthma-related complications and improve the quality of life for affected children. Without proper intervention, the burden of childhood asthma in these settings is likely to remain high, perpetuating cycles of poor health and limited access to care. Addressing these barriers and providing caregivers with the knowledge and resources they need is essential for improving asthma outcomes in low-resource environments.

3. Challenges in diagnosing and managing childhood asthma

The signs and symptoms of asthma can differ significantly from child to child and may fluctuate as they grow older [15]. In very young children, the most common symptoms of asthma include recurrent coughing, wheezing—a high-pitched, whistle-like sound produced during exhalation—shortness of breath, and a sensation of tightness or discomfort in the chest. Although, studies show that most children exhibit symptoms of asthma before the age of 5 [13]. However, diagnosing asthma in very young children, such as preschoolers, presents significant challenges due to the complexity of the disease's underlying pathogenesis. This complexity often makes it difficult for caregivers and even doctors to recognize asthma symptoms at such an early age [16, 17].

Various studies have established the existence of multiple asthma phenotypes, which can complicate both diagnosis and treatment strategies [17]. The most common clinical phenotypes of asthma include atopic asthma, which is more frequently observed in school-aged children, and episodic viral wheeze, which is more common in preschoolers [16]. It is uncertain whether children who wheeze during severe colds or respiratory infections will later develop asthma [18]. In many cases, the first signs of asthma in young children manifest as recurrent wheezing, often triggered by respiratory viruses [19, 20]. Wheezing, however, remains a poorly understood symptom, as caregivers often struggle to differentiate whether it is caused by asthma or another respiratory or atopic condition. Given that several other conditions can cause recurrent wheezing in young children, medical examinations and clinical tests to measure lung function are recommended for a proper diagnosis of asthma.

Researchers have pointed out the difficulty, and sometimes the impossibility, of diagnosing asthma in children under the age of 5 [16]. This age group, including infants and toddlers, tends to have smaller and narrower bronchial tubes, making them more susceptible to colds and respiratory infections. Additionally, children in this age group may not be able to complete airflow tests that are essential for measuring lung function. These tests, such as spirometry, require blowing forcefully into a device, which can be challenging for young children who cannot blow out as hard and quickly as required [15]. As a result, asthma diagnosis in preschoolers is often delayed until after months or even years of observing symptoms.

In contrast, children above the age of 5 can be diagnosed using the same tests that are used for adults, such as lung function tests (spirometry) to measure airflow. However, for preschool-age children or younger, diagnosis is more difficult due to their inability to perform these tests accurately. According to the American College of Allergy, Asthma, and Immunology, some children are not diagnosed with asthma until much later, after prolonged observation of symptoms. Infants and toddlers, being too young to articulate their symptoms, rely on the attentiveness of caregivers to notice signs of asthma [16, 21].

Evidence-based studies comparing asthma in children and adults indicate that, while the disease's pathophysiology may be similar, children face unique challenges, including school absenteeism, limitations in play and sports, hospitalization, and frequent emergency room visits [21, 22]. Despite these challenges, there is no cure for asthma, only preventive measures and treatment plans that help manage the condition and improve the quality of life for children affected by it [13].

Furthermore, childhood asthma has profound psychosocial and economic impacts on millions of children and their families [23]. These impacts include the stress of managing the illness, the cost of healthcare, and the limitations it imposes on children's daily activities [13]. Developing effective management strategies and providing support to both caregivers and healthcare providers is essential to reducing the burden of asthma in children. At the same time, recognizing these symptoms early is crucial, as timely diagnosis and effective management can help reduce the frequency and severity of asthma attacks. Additionally, understanding the unique triggers that exacerbate asthma symptoms, such as allergens, respiratory infections, and environmental pollutants, is essential for caregivers and healthcare providers. This knowledge empowers families to implement preventive strategies, thus improving the overall quality of life for children living with asthma.

4. Exploring caregivers' understanding of childhood asthma triggers in economically disadvantaged areas

Caregivers' knowledge of the common causes of childhood asthma in resource-poor settings often varies based on their education, access to healthcare services, and other social and economic factors. According to Akinso et al. (2023), the knowledge that caregivers have regarding asthma triggers and effective management practices plays a crucial role in determining how well their children's asthma is controlled [24]. Caregivers who are knowledgeable about common asthma triggers—such as allergens, environmental pollutants, respiratory infections, and weather changes—are better equipped to minimize exposure to these triggers. This proactive approach can significantly reduce the frequency and severity of asthma attacks, leading to better overall asthma control [24].

Moreover, caregivers who are informed about proper management practices, including the correct use of medications (such as inhalers and corticosteroids), adherence to prescribed treatment plans, and the importance of regular follow-ups with healthcare providers, are more likely to implement these strategies effectively. Their ability to recognize early warning signs of worsening asthma and respond appropriately can also contribute to better management outcomes [24].

In contrast, caregivers with limited knowledge may inadvertently expose their children to asthma triggers or neglect essential management strategies. This lack of understanding can result in poorly controlled asthma, characterized by frequent symptoms, increased reliance on emergency care, and a negative impact on the child's quality of life, including difficulties in school and recreational activities [24].

Thus, enhancing caregivers' knowledge about asthma triggers and management practices is essential for improving asthma control in children. Targeted education and support programs can empower caregivers to take an active role in managing their children's condition, ultimately leading to better health outcomes.

However, in general, the following factors are typically recognized or misunderstood as causes or triggers of asthma in such settings:

1. Environmental factors

    - *Air pollution:* Exposure to pollutants from traffic, factories, and indoor smoke from cooking with biomass fuels (like wood, coal, and dung) is a well-known cause of asthma.

    - *Dust and allergens:* Poor housing conditions often lead to higher exposure to dust mites, mold, and animal dander, which can exacerbate asthma symptoms.

    - *Tobacco smoke:* Second-hand smoke exposure, especially in households where smoking is prevalent, increases the risk of asthma in children [25].

2. Infections

    - *Respiratory infections:* Viral and bacterial infections such as pneumonia and bronchitis are often seen as major triggers for asthma flare-ups in children. In many cases, caregivers may associate recurrent infections with asthma.

    - *Tuberculosis:* In settings where tuberculosis is prevalent, it may be mistaken for asthma or believed to be a cause of asthma.

3. Weather conditions

    - *Cold air and humidity:* Sudden changes in weather, cold temperatures, and humid environments can trigger asthma symptoms, but caregivers may not always connect these conditions to the cause of asthma.

4. Indoor environmental conditions

    - *Overcrowded living conditions:* Poor ventilation in crowded homes can increase exposure to indoor pollutants and allergens, aggravating asthma symptoms.
    - *Dampness and mold:* Damp environments promote the growth of mold, which can worsen asthma in children.

5. Nutritional factors

    - *Malnutrition:* Undernutrition weakens the immune system and makes children more susceptible to infections that may trigger asthma.
    - *Food allergies:* In some cases, caregivers may be aware of certain foods (e.g., eggs, nuts) triggering asthma or allergic reactions, though this knowledge may be inconsistent.

6. Genetic and hereditary factors

    - Some caregivers may recognize that asthma can run in families, understanding that children with a family history of asthma or allergies are at higher risk.

7. Misconceptions and cultural beliefs

    - *Spiritual or supernatural beliefs:* In some communities, asthma may be misunderstood because of spiritual forces or curses, leading to delayed medical intervention.
    - *Blaming physical activities:* Caregivers might mistakenly believe that physical exertion alone causes asthma, without understanding the underlying chronic condition.

8. Lack of awareness

    - *Limited knowledge of asthma as a chronic disease:* In many low-resource settings, caregivers may not fully understand asthma as a manageable, chronic condition, and may not be aware of preventive measures, such as avoiding specific environmental triggers or adhering to prescribed medications like inhalers.

Efforts to improve caregivers' knowledge through health education campaigns, community health workers, and healthcare provider training can help in better asthma management and prevention in resource-poor settings.

5. Prevention intervention for caregivers: Best practices in diagnosing, treating, and long-term management of childhood asthma

Childhood asthma is a chronic respiratory condition that requires careful diagnosis, treatment, and long-term management. Effective asthma management involves both medical intervention and active caregiver participation. In low-resource settings, like many parts of Nigeria, caregivers often face significant barriers to managing asthma due to a lack of knowledge, access to healthcare, and financial constraints [24]. A well-designed prevention intervention for caregivers focuses on increasing their understanding and ability to manage the disease to reduce exacerbations and improve the quality of life for affected children.

1. *Diagnosing childhood asthma:* Early and accurate diagnosis of asthma is critical in preventing severe asthma exacerbations. Unfortunately, many caregivers may not recognize the symptoms of asthma in young children, and diagnosis can be delayed.

   Best practices

   a. *Education on early symptoms:* Caregivers need to be trained to recognize early asthma symptoms such as persistent coughing, wheezing, shortness of breath, or chest tightness, especially after physical activity or at night. Education on the difference between asthma symptoms and common colds or respiratory infections is essential.

   b. *Regular medical consultations:* Encouraging regular check-ups with healthcare professionals, especially if symptoms are recurring or severe. Since spirometry (lung function testing) may not be possible for children under 5, doctors may rely on symptom history and physical examinations [12].

   c. *Symptom tracking:* Caregivers should keep detailed records of their child's symptoms, frequency of episodes, and any potential triggers, as this information is vital for an accurate diagnosis [26].

2. *Treating childhood asthma:* Treatment focuses on controlling symptoms, preventing exacerbations, and enabling children to lead normal lives. This requires both medication-adherence and awareness of triggers.

   Best practices

   a. *Use of quick-relief and controller medications:* Caregivers need to understand the difference between *quick-relief medications* (e.g., inhaled bronchodilators for immediate symptom relief) and *long-term controller medications* (e.g., inhaled corticosteroids to reduce airway inflammation).

   b. *Proper inhaler technique:* Inhaler technique training is crucial. Poor technique reduces the effectiveness of the treatment. Caregivers should be taught the correct way to administer inhalers, possibly with the use of a spacer, which helps ensure the medication reaches the lungs.

c. *Asthma action plan:* Developing an individualized asthma action plan with a healthcare provider is critical. The plan should outline what to do daily to manage asthma, how to identify worsening symptoms, and when to seek emergency care. Caregivers should have a written, easy-to-follow action plan for their child's asthma management.

d. *Overcoming misconceptions:* Caregivers must be reassured that inhalers are safe, non-addictive, and crucial for managing asthma. Public health campaigns can be employed to dispel common myths, such as the belief that asthma medications stunt growth or are harmful in the long term.

3. Long-term management of childhood asthma: Asthma is a long-term condition that requires ongoing monitoring and adjustments in treatment as the child grows and changes

   Best practices

   a. *Avoidance of triggers:* Caregivers should be educated on common asthma triggers such as dust, pollen, smoke, animal dander, cold air, and respiratory infections. They need to be trained on how to minimize their child's exposure to these triggers. For instance, keeping the home dust-free, avoiding second-hand smoke, and controlling allergens can significantly reduce the frequency of asthma attacks.

   b. *Monitoring for exacerbations:* Regularly assessing asthma control is essential. Caregivers should look out for signs that their child's asthma is not well-controlled, such as increased use of quick-relief medication, frequent nighttime symptoms, or limited physical activity.

   c. *School and physical activity:* Ensuring that children can participate in school and physical activities is important for their overall well-being. Caregivers should work with teachers and school staff to ensure that the child has access to their medication and an asthma action plan during school hours.

   d. *Regular follow-ups with healthcare providers:* Regular check-ups help monitor the child's growth and development, and healthcare providers can adjust treatment plans based on changing symptoms or needs.

4. *Empowering caregivers:* Caregivers are at the heart of effective asthma management. A key intervention focus should be building their confidence and knowledge in managing asthma daily.

   Best practices

   a. *Asthma education programs:* Community-based or healthcare-based asthma education programs for caregivers can greatly improve knowledge and self-efficacy. Programs can cover asthma basics, symptom management, medication use, and prevention strategies.

   b. *Support networks:* Establishing support groups where caregivers can share experiences, challenges, and strategies for managing asthma can provide emotional support and practical advice.

c. *Access to resources:* Ensuring that caregivers have access to affordable medications, inhalers, and educational materials (in local languages) is essential for ongoing management. Public health systems can provide low-cost or subsidized asthma medications in low-resource areas.

d. *Emergency preparedness:* Caregivers should know when and how to seek emergency care for asthma exacerbations. They must be trained to recognize severe symptoms (e.g., difficulty breathing, blue lips, or face) that require immediate medical attention.

6. Summary

The causes of childhood asthma are diverse and multifaceted, involving a combination of genetic, environmental, socioeconomic, and lifestyle factors. Although asthma can affect children from various regions and backgrounds, certain causes and risk factors significantly contribute to its prevalence across the globe. While asthma affects children globally, the burden is disproportionately higher in low- and middle-income countries, where limited access to healthcare and exposure to environmental risk factors pose significant challenges. Understanding the various causes of childhood asthma is crucial for developing targeted interventions that can reduce its prevalence and improve management, particularly in high-burden regions.

Managing asthma in children is particularly challenging due to the complexity of the disease and its varied manifestations. Effective asthma management begins with a proper understanding of the disease, including the recognition of early symptoms and potential triggers, frequent monitoring, and adherence to prescribed medications. Caregivers play a vital role in this process, particularly in ensuring the appropriate use of quick-relief medications and preventive treatments. For children with asthma in resource-poor settings, the role of caregivers is crucial in managing the disease. By focusing on early diagnosis, appropriate treatment, long-term management, and empowering caregivers through education, childhood asthma outcomes can be significantly improved. Public health interventions should prioritize caregiver education, access to affordable treatments, and support systems to ensure that children with asthma lead healthy, active lives despite their condition.

7. Case studies

Case Study 1: Asthma in preschool-age children in Southwest Nigeria.

7.1 Case summary

Fola is a 4-year-old girl, a pre-schooler living in a rural area of Ilesha with her parents and two siblings. Her family lives in a one-bedroom home with poor ventilation and limited access to healthcare. Fola has been diagnosed with mild intermittent asthma, a condition her parents struggle to manage due to a lack of access to asthma

DOI: http://dx.doi.org/10.5772/intechopen.1008341

education and medication. Her parents have noticed that Fola's asthma worsens when she plays outside in a dusty environment or when there is smoke from nearby wood-burning stoves.

In the past 6 months, Fola has visited the emergency room three times due to severe asthma attacks. Her parents report that these attacks are often triggered by exposure to dust and fumes, particularly when her mother is cooking inside the house. Despite the frequent emergency room visits, Fola's parents are unaware of how to properly manage her asthma at home, and there has been little guidance from healthcare providers in their area.

7.1.1 Discussion questions

1. *Environmental triggers and impact:*

    - What specific measures could be taken to reduce Fola's exposure to environmental triggers at home? Consider the family's rural setting and limited resources.

2. *Severity and management:*

    - Studies have shown that most preschool-age children, including Fola, have mild intermittent asthma. What are the defining characteristics of mild intermittent asthma, and how can caregivers differentiate between mild and severe asthma symptoms in young children?

    - How does the severity of asthma in preschoolers impact the approach to asthma management compared to school-age children?

3. *Socioeconomic and healthcare disparities:*

    - Asthma studies have consistently highlighted the disproportionate impact of asthma on minorities and those of lower socioeconomic status. How might socioeconomic factors, such as housing, education, and access to healthcare, influence asthma outcomes in children like Fola?

    - What role can local healthcare providers play in educating families in low-income communities on managing asthma in children, given the barriers to healthcare access?

4. *Long-term management and preventive strategies:*

    - What are some long-term strategies that could be implemented in low-income countries to improve asthma management for children? Consider community-based interventions, healthcare education, and environmental improvements.

    - How can caregivers be empowered to prevent emergency room visits, and what educational tools or resources could be most effective in rural and low-resource settings?

5. *Policy implications and healthcare access:*

- What policies could be advocated for at the local or national level to reduce the impact of asthma triggers in rural homes? How could these policies improve healthcare access for children with asthma?
- How can healthcare infrastructure in low-income countries be improved to better address chronic conditions like asthma in young children?

Case Study 2: Challenges in diagnosing and managing childhood asthma in low-income countries.

Background: In Nigeria, childhood asthma is a growing public health concern

Background: In sub-Saharan Africa (SSA), childhood asthma is a growing public health concern, especially in rural and low-resource areas. Despite global advances in asthma care and management, many children in SSA experience poorly controlled asthma due to delays in diagnosis, limited access to healthcare, and misconceptions about the disease. Caregivers, often mothers or close family members, play a critical role in managing the condition, yet they face multiple barriers in effectively caring for their children with asthma. These barriers include a lack of awareness about asthma symptoms, inadequate access to healthcare, financial constraints, and widespread misconceptions about the treatment.

7.2 Case summary

Mrs. Conga lives in a rural community in Ghana and cares for her 4-year-old son, Kofi, who has been experiencing recurrent wheezing, coughing, and breathlessness for over a year. She initially thought Kofi's symptoms were due to a recurring cold and treated him with herbal remedies passed down through generations. After several emergency visits to the local clinic, a healthcare provider suggested Kofi might have asthma. Mrs. Conga was unfamiliar with the term and confused about what it meant for her son's health. She was reluctant to use the inhaler prescribed by the clinic due to fears that her son might become addicted to it, as other caregivers in her community warned her.

Over time, Kofi's symptoms worsened. He often missed school and could no longer play with his friends because physical activity triggered his breathing difficulties. Mrs. Conga took him to a larger hospital in the nearby town, but the long distance and high cost of transport made regular visits difficult. At the hospital, a doctor explained that Kofi had asthma, which required long-term management, and prescribed daily medication. However, Mrs. Conga struggled to adhere to the treatment plan due to its cost and her uncertainty about how to correctly administer the inhaler.

7.3 Key challenges

1. *Delay in diagnosis:* Kofi's asthma symptoms were initially misinterpreted as a common cold by both his caregiver and local healthcare providers, leading to delayed diagnosis and treatment.

2. *Misconceptions about asthma and inhalers:* Mrs. Conga had misconceptions about the use of inhalers, believing they could be addictive or harmful in the long term, which affected her willingness to follow the prescribed treatment.

3. *Financial constraints:* The high cost of transportation to the hospital and the long-term expense of medications created significant financial strain for the family, limiting their ability to seek continuous medical care.

4. *Healthcare access:* The rural location of the family's home restricted access to qualified healthcare providers and asthma management resources.

5. *Lack of education:* Mrs. Conga lacked access to accurate information about asthma, its symptoms, and how to manage it effectively, contributing to poor adherence to the treatment plan.

7.4 Discussion questions

1. What are the main barriers faced by caregivers like Mrs. Conga in diagnosing and managing childhood asthma in rural Ghana? *Consider factors such as healthcare access, financial constraints, and knowledge gaps.*

2. How do misconceptions about asthma and its treatment, particularly regarding inhaler use, impact asthma management in resource-limited settings?

3. What roles do cultural beliefs, and traditional practices play in delaying asthma diagnosis and treatment in rural Ghanaian communities?

4. How can healthcare providers and public health initiatives better educate caregivers about asthma and reduce the stigma surrounding inhaler use in low-resource areas?

5. What strategies could be implemented to improve asthma care for children in rural and underserved communities in Ghana? *Consider interventions such as community education programs, mobile health clinics, and subsidized medication.*

6. How can the government and health organizations address the financial barriers that caregivers face in accessing continuous asthma care for their children?

7. In what ways can healthcare systems in developing countries like Ghana adopt asthma management guidelines to meet the specific challenges faced by caregivers in rural settings?

7.5 Definition of terms

- *Airways:* A child's airways bring air-containing oxygen into the lungs and expel carbon dioxide. These include the nose, mouth, voice box (larynx), windpipe (trachea), and bronchial tubes in the lungs. In asthma, the airways can become tightened, blocked, or inflamed, causing breathing difficulties.

- *Allergens:* Substances capable of causing an allergic reaction. Common allergens include dust mites, pollen, pet dander, insect venom, mold, certain medications, and various foods.
- *Allergy:* A reaction where a child's immune system overreacts to certain substances like dust mites, pollen, pets, or specific foods. Symptoms can include wheezing, coughing, swelling, rashes, itching, or sneezing. Allergic reactions can also trigger asthma symptoms.
- *Asthma:* A chronic respiratory condition that causes the airways to narrow and become inflamed. This leads to difficulty in breathing and triggers symptoms like coughing, wheezing, chest tightness, and shortness of breath.
- *Asthma action plan:* A personalized treatment plan developed with a healthcare professional to help caregivers manage and control their child's asthma. The plan outlines daily medication routines, monitors symptoms, and provides instructions for early treatment if asthma worsens.
- *Asthma exacerbation:* Also known as an asthma attack, this occurs when a child's asthma symptoms (coughing, wheezing, breathlessness, and tightness in the chest) worsen and require quick-relief medication, such as an inhaler, for better control.
- *Asthma symptoms:* The physical signs of asthma include coughing, wheezing, chest tightness, and shortness of breath.
- *Poorly controlled asthma:* Asthma, that is not well managed due to exposure to allergens, failure to adhere to prescribed preventive measures, or missing medication doses as advised by a healthcare professional.
- *Healthcare professional:* A trained medical expert capable of diagnosing, treating, and advising on health conditions. Examples include doctors, asthma specialists, nurses, midwives, and pharmacists.
- *Inflammation:* Redness and swelling in body tissues. In asthma, inflammation occurs in the lungs, leading to symptoms such as coughing, wheezing, and breathlessness, and can trigger asthma attacks.
- *Reliever:* An asthma inhaler used to quickly alleviate asthma symptoms during an attack. Relievers help relax the airways, making it easier for the child to breathe after an asthma episode.
- *Severe asthma:* A form of asthma that does not respond to regular medications and requires specialized care from healthcare professionals to manage the condition.
- *Side effects:* Unwanted reactions to asthma medications, especially when used without medical supervision or not following the instructions on the medication leaflet.
- *Trigger:* Any condition or activity that worsens a child's asthma symptoms. A child may have multiple triggers.
- *Wheeze:* A high-pitched, whistling sound made when breathing. It is often a sign that the child's asthma is not well controlled.

Acknowledgements

I would like to extend my heartfelt gratitude to all those who contributed to the completion of this chapter. A special thank you to my supervisor Dr. Atin Adhikari, at Georgia Southern University, whose guidance, support, and expertise were instrumental in shaping the direction of this work. Your mentorship has been invaluable, and I am deeply appreciative of the time and knowledge you have shared with me.

I am also grateful for the experiences I gained while working with the Ministry of Health and various NGOs in Nigeria. These experiences have shaped my understanding of public health challenges in resource-limited settings and have deeply influenced my perspective on the importance of equitable healthcare access. The knowledge and skills I acquired during this time continue to guide my approach to global health education and research, particularly in addressing the needs of underserved populations. To the caregivers and healthcare providers in the rural parts of Nigeria who shared their experiences—your challenges and dedication inspired much of the content and remain a constant reminder of the crucial role caregivers play in managing childhood asthma.

Additionally, I would like to acknowledge the unwavering support of my family, the Akinso family, especially my daughter Oluwatamilore, who provided constant encouragement throughout this journey. Finally, I extend my gratitude to my students, whose enthusiasm for global health continues to inspire my work.

This chapter is dedicated to all those working to improve the lives of children with asthma, particularly in underserved communities. Your efforts are deeply appreciated.

Portions of this chapter were previously published in the doctoral thesis by the same author, Oyindamola Akinso, titled *Childhood Asthma Management Practices in Rural Nigeria: Exploring the Knowledge, Attitude, and Practice of Caregivers in Oyo State* (2020). This unpublished doctoral thesis was submitted to the Jiann-Ping Hsu College of Public Health, Georgia Southern University, and is available from the Georgia Southern University digital repository. Available from: [https://scholars.georgiasouthern.edu/en/publications/childhood-asthma-management-practices-in-rural-nigeria-exploring–11].

In accordance with the guidelines IntechOpen, I acknowledge the use of AI tool (ChatGPT by OpenAI) for language polishing of the manuscript. I confirm that the tool was used in the preparation of this manuscript, specifically to assist with language editing, and organizing references. I take full responsibility for the content and affirm that the manuscript adheres to all publication ethics standards.

Conflict of interest

The authors declare no conflict of interest.

Acronyms and abbreviations

AAAI	American Academy of Allergy, Asthma, & Immunology
AAPs	asthma action plans
AKQ	asthma knowledge questionnaire

ASSIA	applied social sciences index & abstracts
CARAT	child asthma risk assessment tool
CDC	centers for disease control and prevention
CINAHL	the cumulative index to nursing and allied health literature
FGDs	focus group discussions
HCPs	health care providers
IRB	The Institutional Review Board
ISAAC	The International Study of Asthma and Allergies in Childhood
NAEPP	National Asthma Education and Prevention Program
NHIS	National Health Insurance Scheme
NHLBI	National Heart, Lung, and Blood Institute
NGO	nongovernmental organization
WHO	world health organization

Author details

Oyindamola Akinso
Wingate University, North Carolina, United States of America

*Address all correspondence to: o.soremekun@wingate.edu

References

[1] Akhiwu HO, Asani MO, Johnson AB, Ibrahim M. Epidemiology of pediatric asthma in a Nigerian population. Journal of the Health Research and Reviews. 2017;**4**(3):130

[2] Desalu OO, Onyedum CC, Iseh KR, Salawu FK, Salami AK. Asthma in Nigeria: Are the facilities and resources available to support internationally endorsed standards of care? Health Policy. 2011;**99**(3):250-254

[3] AlOtaibi E, AlAteeq M. Knowledge and practice of parents and guardians about childhood asthma at king Abdulaziz Medical City for National Guard, Riyadh, Saudi Arabia. Risk Management and Healthcare Policy. 2018;**11**:67

[4] World Health Organization. Asthma: Key Facts. Geneva, Switzerland: WHO; 2017. Available from: https://www.who.int/news-room/fact-sheets/detail/asthma [Accessed: February 11, 2018]

[5] Mallol J. Childhood asthma in developing countries: Low-income aspects and related matters. Allergologia et Immunopathologia. 2000;**28**(5):283-286

[6] Kuti BP, Omole KO, Kuti DK. Factors associated with childhood asthma control in a resource-poor center. Journal of Family Medicine and Primary Care. 2017;**6**(2):222

[7] Kuti BP, Omole KO. Epidemiology, triggers, and severity of childhood asthma in Ilesa, Nigeria: Implications for management and control. Nigerian Medical Journal. 2017;**58**(1):13

[8] Shimwela M, Mwita JC, Mwandri M, Rwegerera GM, Mashalla Y, Mugusi F. Asthma prevalence, knowledge, and perceptions among secondary school pupils in rural and urban coastal districts in Tanzania. BMC Public Health. 2014;**14**(1):387

[9] Kuti BP, Omole KO. Factors associated with caregivers' knowledge about childhood asthma in Ilesa, Nigeria. Annals of Nigerian Medicine. 2016;**10**(1):30

[10] Marsden EJ, Somwe SW, Chabala C, Soriano JB, Vallès CP, Anchochea J. Knowledge and perceptions of asthma in Zambia: A cross-sectional survey. BMC Pulmonary Medicine. 2016;**16**(1):33

[11] Bellin MH, Land C, Newsome A, Kub J, Mudd SS, Bollinger ME, et al. Caregiver perception of asthma management of children in the context of poverty. The Journal of Asthma. 2017;**54**(2):162-172

[12] Mayo Clinic. Treating asthma in children under 5. Mayo clinic. 2019. Available from: https://www.mayoclinic.org/diseases-conditions/childhood-asthma/in-depth/asthma-in-children/art-20044376 [Accessed: March 20, 2020]

[13] American Academy of Allergy, Asthma & Immunology. Childhood Asthma Definition. Milwaukee, Wisconsin, USA: AAAAI; 2018. Available from: https://www.aaaai.org/conditions-and-treatments/conditions-dictionary/Childhood-(pediatric)-Asthma [Accessed: June 12, 2018]

[14] Reyna ME, Dai R, Tran M, Breton V, Medeleanu M, Lou WYW, et al. Development of the childhood asthma risk tool (CHART): A symptom-based tool for screening children at high risk of preschool asthma. Journal of the American Medical Association. 2022. Research report

[15] American College of Allergy, Asthma, and Immunology. Asthma in Children: Overview. IL, USA: ACAAI; 2014. Available from: https://acaai.org/asthma/who-has-asthma/children [Accessed: June 12, 2018]

[16] Townshend J, Hails S, McKean M. Diagnosis of asthma in children. BMJ. 2007;**335**(7612):198-202

[17] SWSD. Multiple Phenotypes of Asthma Can Coexist. Philadelphia, Pennsylvania, USA: Health Union, LLC; 2017. Available from: https://asthma.net/living/multiple-phenotypes-of-asthma-can-co-exist [Accessed: December 7, 2018]

[18] Ng MCW, How CH. Recurrent wheeze and cough in young children: Is it asthma? Singapore Medical Journal. 2014;**55**(5):236

[19] van Aalderen WM. Childhood asthma: Diagnosis and treatment. Cairo: Scientifica; 2012

[20] Bhatia R. Wheezing and Asthma in Infants and Young Children: Merck Manuals. Rahway, New Jersey, USA: Merck & Co., Inc.; 2018. Available from: https://www.merckmanuals.com/professional/pediatrics/respiratory-disorders-in-young-children/wheezing-and-asthma-in-infants-and-young-children [Accessed: December 7, 2018]

[21] Mayo Clinic. Childhood Asthma: Diagnosis and Treatment. Rochester, Minnesota: Mayo Clinic; 2018. Available from: https://www.mayoclinic.org/diseases-conditions/childhood-asthma/symptoms-causes/syc-20351507 [Accessed: November 15, 2018]

[22] Johnson SB, Spin P, Connolly F, Stein M, Cheng TL, Connor K. Asthma and attendance in urban schools. Preventing Chronic Disease. 2019;**16**. Available from: https://www.cdc.gov/pcd/issues/2019/19_0074.htm

[23] Rastogi D, Madhok N, Kipperman S. Caregiver asthma knowledge, aptitude, and practice in high healthcare utilizing children: Effect of an educational intervention. Pediatric Allergy, Immunology and Pulmonology. 2013;**26** (3):128-139

[24] Akinso O, Adhikari A, Yin J, Chopak-Foss J, Shah G. Childhood asthma management practices in rural Nigeria: Exploring the knowledge, attitude, and practice of caregivers in Oyo state. Children. 2023;**10**(6):1043. DOI: 10.3390/children10061043

[25] Ganesh B, Skopec CPSL, Zhu J. The Relationship between Housing and Asthma among School-Age Children. Washington, D.C., USA: Urban Institute; 2017. Research Report

[26] Falade AG, Olawuyi JF, Osinusi K, Onadeko BO. Prevalence and severity of symptoms of asthma, allergic rhinoconjunctivitis, and atopic eczema in 6-7-year-old Nigerian primary school children: The international study of asthma and allergies in childhood. Medical Principles and Practice. 2004;**13**: 20-25. DOI: 10.1159/000074036

Chapter 2

Common Immunopathogenesis of Three Pediatric Chronic Lung Disorders

Terry Chin

Abstract

The epithelial cells lining the airways serve as a physical barrier to various external potential injurious agents. Therefore, injury to the epithelial layer results in an immunological reaction to protect the body from infections and other potential toxins. However, these processes can also lead to deleterious effects if the injury is continuous and/or extreme and therefore result in disorders such as asthma and other chronic lung diseases. This chapter will review the potential immunopathogenesis of three childhood lung diseases: asthma, neonatal chronic bronchopulmonary dysplasia (BPD) and cystic fibrosis (CF). Asthma is one of the most common chronic respiratory diseases in both adults and children. Although BPD and CF are not as common both are a source of significant morbidity and mortality and requires not a small amount of resources to manage and treat. Specifically, it will review evidence showing that there is production of various cytokines by epithelial (and other immune cells in the lung) as well as an influx of inflammatory cells upon exposure to various materials such as gas and particles from car emissions, tobacco smoke, pathogens and various allergens such as pollens and animal dander. It will attempt to correlate the pathology with current therapy and suggest future treatment options.

Keywords: airway epithelium, epithelial cells, cytokines, asthma, bronchopyulmonary dysplasia, cystic fibrosis

1. Introduction

As cells lining the respiratory tract from the nasal opening to the interior of the lung, the airway epithelium serves varying functions. Its main goal is to allow the exchange of gases. However, that also makes the host very susceptible to many substances in the inhaled air with potential pathogens such as microbial organisms and other injurious agents such as allergens and air pollutants. Therefore, airway epithelial cells (AECs) have developed numerous strategies to combat these external factors. There exists a physical barrier to prevent entry of these potential harmful substances. Certain AECs can produce mucus to trap these particles, other cells secrete chemicals to neutralize any toxins or microbial pathogens or mediators to activate the innate immune cells present or recruit other immune cells to fight the infection. This release of mediators results in an inflammatory reaction in the airways which can also be deleterious and play a role in several disorders. This chapter will review how this epithelial response plays a role in three common childhood lung diseases: asthma, neonatal chronic bronchopulmonary dysplasia (BPD) and cystic fibrosis (ICF). Understanding the underlying immunopathogenesis in these conditions will also enable one to appreciate the mechanisms of therapeutic interventions currently and potentially in the future.

2. Functions of the airway epithelium

2.1 The epithelial layer of the airways serves as a physical barrier

The nasal airway epithelium is composed of several types of cells, including columnar epithelial and secretory or goblet cells which overlie the basal cells, which are progenitor cells. As the airways extend into the lungs and branch into bronchial tubes, the epithelial cells differentiate into highly specialized cells becoming cuboidal in shape and eventually flattened into simple squamous pneumocytes in the alveoli (alveolar type 1 or AT-1 cells). Throughout the airways the entire epithelial sheet serves as a physical barrier limiting access to the internal milieu of the body. This is due to the presence of cell-to-cell adhesion structures at the apical ends of the epithelial cells. These tight junctions are formed by three different transmembrane and intracellular proteins (junctional adhesion molecules or JAM, occludin and claudin) which are joined to the intracellular actin cytoskeleton by corresponding cytoplasmic scaffolding proteins ZO-1, 2 and 3, respectively, creating a perijunctional actin belt. The cellular sheet and belt is given further support by adherens junctions (AJs) and desmosomes. AJs consist of the transmembrane protein E-cadherin and intracellular components (p120-catenin, α-catenin, β-catenin) linking to actin to further enhance the strength of the sheet [1]. Finally, desmosomes (also known as macula adherens) are stronger than AJs due to their connection to the intracellular intermediate filament network and cellular cytoskeleton. They connect cell-to-cell but also cell to the basement membrane via hemi-desmosomes. Their anchor proteins (desmoglein, desmocollin) bind to integrin proteins either on adjacent cells or other structures such as the basement membrane or basal lamina. The membrane is comprised of matrix with laminin, fibronectin, heparin sulfate proteoglycans and collagen network and serves to maintain the epithelial structure and orientation. Therefore the entire network of tight junctions and AJs serve as an impermeable sheet with desmosomes and hemi-desmosomes giving the sheet structure strength and aids in resisting shearing forces. As shown in **Figure 1**, this epithelial sheet prevents particulate matter, noxious gases and pathogens from entering inside the host. It also serves to prevent or limit fluid loss by regulating movement of ions and fluids.

2.2 The epithelial layer also produces a chemical barrier

The development of ciliated and goblet cells from the basal cells involves activation and expression of various transcription factors and proteins giving rise to an

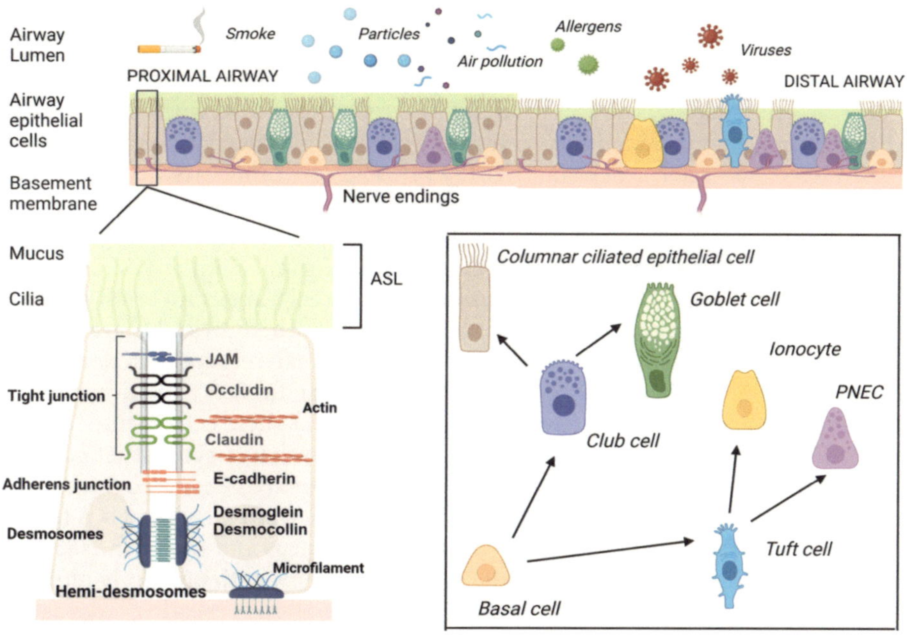

Figure 1.
The cellular barrier function of the respiratory epithelium. The cells are linked by three different physical attachments (tight junction, adherens junction and desmosomes). Specifically, components of tight junction (junctional adhesion molecules or JAM, occludin and claudin) are attached to actin fibers forming a perijunctional actin belt. This cellular sheet is further strengthened two other attachments: adherens junctions with its protein E-cadherin also attached to actin and desmosomes with its components desmoglein and desmocollin joined to microfilaments. Half of the desmosome complex (hemi-desmosome) attach to the basement membrane via anchor proteins, thus strengthening the cellular sheet and creating a cellular barrier in preventing penetration of luminal particles such as allergens, microbial organisms such as viruses, and airway irritants from inhaled air containing pollution and/or smoke. Note that part of the epithelium are also nerve fibers enabling sensory perception of conditions in the airway lumen from certain specialized AECs. The insert depicts the differentiation of the various epithelial cell types from the basal cells, which are the principal stem cells of the airways. Each of these cells has unique immunologic as well as sensory functions in providing a chemical barrier. Mucus is produced by goblet cells and can entrap inhaled particles and allergens. Cilia from columnar ciliated cells move the mucus containing fluid on their apical surface from distal parts of the airway to proximal location where the contents can be coughed out. Pulmonary neuroendocrine cells (PNECs) can influence mucus production and also have the ability to function as sensory cells within the airways due to their innervation and ability to secrete granules with neurotransmitters. Tuft cells also have apical microvilli on the apical surface with some sensory function. Finally, ionocytes regulate the water and ionic content of fluid in the air surface layer (ASL) through transmembrane channel proteins. Created with BioRender.com.

intermediate cell, club or Clara cell [2] as seen in the insert in **Figure 1**. One set of gene activation (including Notch signaling) then differentiates these cells toward cilia formation, whose rhythmic movement across the epithelial layer moves mucus and any trapped particles up the airways where it can be coughed out of the body or/and swallowed in a process termed mucociliary clearance (MCC). Another set of gene activation cascade results in mucin production (primarily MUC5AC and MUC5B) and the development of a goblet-like cellular appearance (hence their name "goblet cells"). Both club and goblet cells produce mucus. Three rare cell types have other functions in the epithelium [3]. Pulmonary ionocytes comprising about 1% of total AECs significantly influence the composition of the mucus layer by having a majority of the activity of the cystic fibrosis transmembrane conductance regulator

(CFTR) which control ion transport across the apical cell membrane and airway lumen. Pulmonary neuroendocrine cells (PNECs) comprising less than 0.5% of total AECs can influence mucus production by being able to regulate immune response to allergens as well as having the ability to function as sensory cells within the airways due to their innervation and ability to secrete granules with neurotransmitters such as calcintonin-gene-related peptide (CGRP) [4]. They are innervated by sensory (or afferent) and motor (or efferent) nerve fibers. Therefore, they are uniquely capable of receiving nerve signals as well as giving them out through proteins such as CGRP. Similarly, tuft cells have microtubule structures forming apical microvilli on the airway surface enabling some sensory function. These cells are more often seen in gastrointestinal tract but are rarely seen in the airway epithelium and also are thought to be progenitor cells to PNECs and ionocytes [5]. They can secrete both immune mediators (such as interleukin 25 or IL-25 and prostaglandin D2) as well as the neurotransmitter acetylcholine (Ach). The importance of these cells in understanding the relationship between airway epithelium and the network of sympathetic, parasympathetic and sensory nerves in the subepithelial layer are being recognized [6]. The sheet of fluid covering the luminal surface of the airway epithelium is referred to as the airway surface liquid (ASL) and contains both mucus and fluid. The secreted mucin glycoproteins are large heavily glycosylated proteins with tandemly repeating sequences of amino acids with linkage sites via disulfide bonds creating large carbohydrate structures capable of trapping particulate matter and other substances in the inhaled air. The ASL not only contains these secreted gel-forming mucins but also electrolytes via transmembrane ion-channels, anti-microbial products (such as defensins, lysozyme and LL-37) and antioxidants which suppress bacterial growth and can have anti-viral activity. AECs transport secretory immunoglobulin A (IgA) into the airway lumen. It is the presence of these factors in the ASL and the activity of MCC that creates a chemical barrier. The fluid composition of ASL fluctuates depending on other factors such as the body's overall fluid balance with dehydration resulting in a more viscous fluid with hypertonicity.

Morphology of the airway epithelial cells (AECs) changes depending on the airway. The nasal cavity is lined by stratified squamous epithelium, the conducting airways are mainly pseudostratified columnar, ciliated epithelium; the small airways are coated with simple cuboidal AEC; and finally two epithelial cell types exists (thin, elongated type 1 pneumocytes (AT-1) for gas exchange and cuboidal type II pneumocytes (AT-2)) to maintain alveolar patency by secreting surfactant. Here the ASL is very thin layer of surfactant without mucin. Therefore, the physical and chemical barriers extend throughout the respiratory system, both upper and lower respiratory tracts. It should be noted that AT-2 cells have some progenitor capability and can convert to AT-1 cells [7].

2.3 The epithelial layer has immunological functions

Airway epithelial cells (AECs) also engage in host defenses by producing immunological cytokines such as interferon (IFN) which induce other cells to inhibit viral replication as well as recruiting and activating other immune cells to recognize and destroy viral-infected cells. The production of other antimicrobial factors such as defensin, cathelicidin, lactoferrin, lysozyme, and secretory leukocyte proteinase inhibitor (SLPI) help in combating various infections. These factors mediate bacterial killing through different mechanisms. AECs have surface receptors such as Toll-like receptor (TLR) or pathogen-associated receptor (PAR) that can bind to various

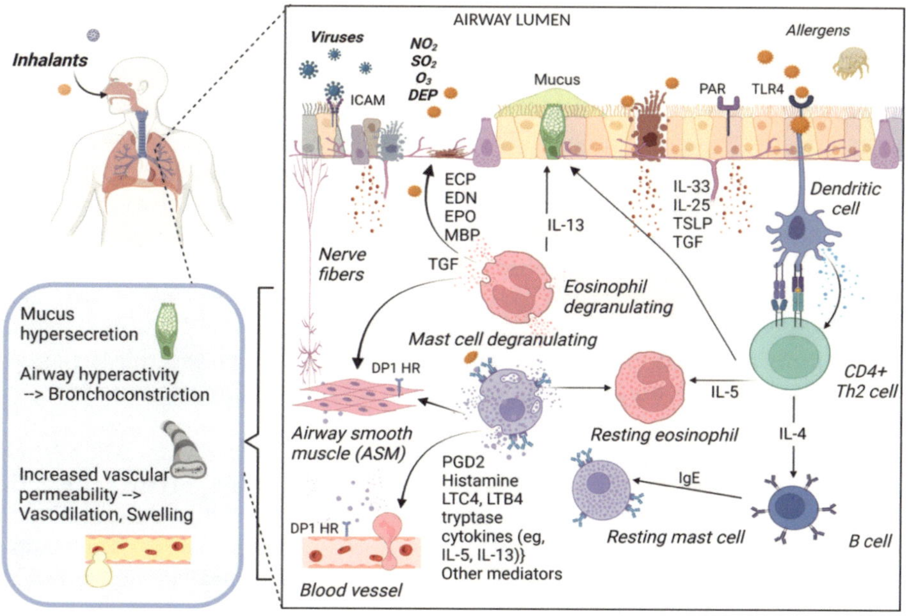

Figure 2.
The key role of epithelial cell in the immunopathogenesis in asthma resulting in its symptoms and signs. Shown in the left insert are three hallmarks of asthma: mucus hypersecretion, airway hyperactivity resulting in bronchoconstriction, and vasodilation with swelling from increased vascular permeability. Increased mucus production from goblet cells is the result of various cytokines (especially IL-13) and nerve innervation. Smooth muscle contraction resulting in bronchial narrowing can be the result of stimulation of receptors (such as histamine receptor or HR or type 1 prostaglandin D2 [PGD2] receptor or DP1) on airway smooth muscle (ASM) cell surface or nerve innervation. Increased vascular permeability is the result of mediators binding to HR or DP1 receptors resulting in increased leakage by endothelial cells. The most common source for IL-13 is Th2 helper cells, but significant amounts can also be produced by eosinophils, mast cells, and other lymphocytes. Mast cell involvement is shown with degranulation occurring with coupling of IgE with allergen resulting in the release of other mediators including PGD2, leukotrienes and histamine; thereby accounting for the immediate allergic asthma response. IgE production is regulated by IL-4 produced by Th2 cells after the allergen is processed by dendritic cells and presented via T cell receptors. Recruitment and activation of eosinophils occurs with PGD2 and IL-5 and their degranulation releases numerous proteins which are toxic to AECs and their cytokines influence ASM. Denudation of AECs exposes nerve fibers resulting in increased AHR. Destruction by AECs can also occur by respiratory viruses binding to receptors such as ICAM and subsequent viral replication inside the cells. Additionally pollutants such as diesel exhaust particles (DEP) and chemicals such as ozone (O_3) result in AEC injury and/or breakdown of tight junctions, allowing for increased entry of allergens and other injurious agents and continuing the inflammatory cycle in both allergic and non-allergic asthma, Created with BioRender.com.

components of bacteria and virus which in turn result in the production of mediators termed alarmins such as thymic stromal lymphopoietin (TSLP) and interleukins 25 (IL-25) and 33 (IL-33). Each of these belongs to a different cytokine family (TSLP to IL-2, IL-25 to IL-17, and IL-33 to IL-1) and contributes to the immune defenses by activating helper T lymphocytes and inducing T2 cytokine secretion and allergic inflammation. These eventually result in the mucus production and eosinophilia typically seen in asthma as shown in **Figure 2** and will be discussed in more detailed below. Interleukin-8 (IL-8) recruits other immune cells such as phagocytic white blood cells (neutrophils) to enter the epithelium to fight pathogens such as bacteria. Neutrophilic inflammation is also enhanced by IL-17. Finally other proinflammatory cytokines produced by epithelial cells also include IL-6, IL-1β, tumor necrosis factor-alpha (TNF-α), interferon-gamma (IFN-γ), granulocyte-macrophage coloncy stimulating factor (GM-CSF). TNF-α and IFN-γ are indicative of T1 cytokine activity or type 1 inflammation involving the cellular immune system. However, anti-inflammatory mediators such as interleukin 10 (IL-10) are also released by AECs and can also result with immunosuppression. Club cells secrete the anti-inflammatory protein uteroglobin (also known as Clara cell protein (CC10, CC16)) which has inhibitory effects on neutrophil and monocyte chemotaxis and production of TNF-α, IFN-γ and IL-1. Uteroglobin levels are decreased in asthma patients; and increased airway hyperactivity (AHR) can be seen in mouse models with reduced uteroglobin levels. Therefore, airway epithelial cells play a central role in the innate immunity as well as down-regulating the immune response so that the airways can repair itself ("remodeling") and limiting bystander cellular damage. Indeed, transforming growth factor beta (TGF-β) released by AEC not only modulates both innate and adaptive immune responses but also can suppress inflammation. Finally, it also plays a role in tissue repair by regulating fibroblast and mesenchymal stem cell (MSC) activity and differentiation.

There is increasing recognition that the interaction between certain AECs (such as PNEC and Tuft), immune cells in the airway and neurons are important in detecting and reacting to potential harmful inhalants. This recognition is due to the ability of these cells to sense the noxious presence within the respiratory tract and then communicate with immune and neural systems to eliminate or neutralize the stimuli. These interactions are mediated by inflammatory cytokines, neurotrophins and neuropeptides. The cough reflex is a well-known protective mechanism to rid the airway of irritants but the precise elucidation of the underlying neural circuitry is not yet known [8]. Ach does induce smooth muscle contraction and bronchial constriction to preventing further insults from entering the distal airways. It also results in increase mucus secretion from the secretory cells. There are other connections to the vascular system and therefore involvement in the regulation of blood flow. Finally, there are neuroimmune pathways that can result in airway neurogenic inflammation [9]. Therefore, its role to chronic inflammatory disorders in the respiratory tract is important to understand.

Finally, the cell death itself can generate a response by innate immune cells [10]. Dying epithelial cells and cell corpses in response to injury also release a set of cytokines initiating innate immune response. This release does not require contact of external elements to cellular receptors.

3. Asthma

The Global Initiative for Asthma (GINA) defines asthma as "a heterogeneous disease, usually characterized by chronic airway inflammation. It is defined by the history of respiratory symptoms, such as wheeze, shortness of breath, chest tightness, and cough that vary over time and in intensity, together with variable expiratory airflow limitation" [11]. It is the heterogeneous nature of the disease that has resulted in current attempts to correlate its various phenotypes on the basis of the underlying immunopathology and to define specific "endotypes" [12, 13]. Recognition of the key role for the Th-2 lymphocyte with its production of IL-4, IL-5, and IL-13 in promoting a proinflammatory eosinophilic state has resulted in the identification of Th2 type asthma. However, identification of other cells (such as dendritic cells) producing these cytokines lead to the current terminology of the type 2 (T2)-high asthma endotype which incorporate both eosinophilic and allergic asthma, which are the most common types seen in children. These patients, who frequently have other manifestations of allergies (such as allergic rhinitis), show increased numbers of IgE and eosinophils in the blood as well as in bronchial biopsies or BAL fluid and elevated levels of IL-4, IL-5, and/or IL-13 protein or mRNA transcripts.

In both human studies and animal models the inhalation of an allergen to which the subject has been sensitized induces airway narrowing and physiologic changes in pulmonary function which are typical of asthma [14]. The changes are similar to other allergic responses at other locations (such as allergic rhinitis or conjunctivitis) where there is an immediate response with exposure to an allergen with release of mediators and then often a delayed reaction characterized by inflammatory cells [15]. It has been shown that the immediate asthmatic response is due to the release of specific mediators from mast cells upon coupling of the allergen to its specific IgE bound on its cell surface as shown in **Figure 2**.

Of the approximate 390 mediators secreted from mast cells [16] the main ones include prostaglandins (especially prostaglandin D2 or PGD2), histamine, leukotrienes (LTC4 and LTB4), cytokines, and serotonin. PGD2 binds to the type 1 prostaglandin D2 (DP1) receptors while histamine binds to H1 receptors (HR) on airway smooth muscle (ASM) and capillary endothelial cells with bronchoconstriction and vasodilation with plasma extravasation with swelling. These two effects result in immediate narrowing of the airways. Additionally, goblet cells respond to PGD2 and LTC4 with increased production of mucus within the airways causing further obstruction. Measurements of airway flow will show an immediate drop in forced expiratory volume in 1 second (FEV_1) as well as peak expiratory flow (PEF) and increase in airway resistance (Raw). Medications which block mast cell degranulation (such as sodium cromolyn and nedocromil) inhibit this early asthmatic response. The decrease in lung function is reversible with bronchodilators, which has been an integral part of the clinical definition of asthma (reversible bronchospasm). Bronchoconstriction results and reaches a maximum within 30 minutes and resolves after 1–3 hours. Further support for the role of these mediators is seen by the increased levels of histamine and leukotrienes in bronchoalveolar lavage (BAL) fluid and urine of subjects taken during this time period. Leukotriene receptor antagonists (LTRAs) or anti-histamine antagonist will also attenuate the pulmonary function drop by about 50%.

This early asthmatic (or allergic) response (EAR) is then followed by a second episode of bronchoconstriction in about 60% of adults and 80% of children after 3–4 hours and reaches a maximum over 6–12 hours [8]. This late asthmatic (allergic) response (LAR) appears to be allergen specific since some allergens such as house dust mite (HDM) and cat allergen are more common than others (such as grass pollen) in resulting in LAR. However, there is no airway inflammation unless exposed to low-dose allergen challenge daily over 5–7 days. Increased airway hyperactivity (AHR) is also seen during the LAR and some have correlated the presence of AHR with airway inflammation [17].

The inhaled allergen activates TLR-4 receptors on epithelial cells (see **Figure 2**), resulting in secretion of IL-25, IL-33 and TSLP (alarmins) all of which induce and enhance the CD4 positive T helper 2 (Th2) lymphocyte and innate lymphoid cells type 2 (ILC2) to secrete IL-4, IL-5 and IL-13 in enhancing IgE production and eosinophil involvement. Alarmins can also stimulate goblet cell production and therefore mucus hypersecretion, which is a feature of asthma. TSLP has multiple effects on mast cells with induction of other cytokines such as IL-5 and IL-13. IL-5 is the key cytokine which mobilizes eosinophils from the bone marrow and promotes their activation, proliferation and increases their survival. It is not surprising then that experimental animal models without the IL-5 gene did not have eosinophilic airway inflammation. Other chemo-attractants are also produced resulting in increased dendritic cells in the sub-epithelial layer where they process allergens and act as antigen-presenting cells to CD4 lymphocytes. The net effect is production of allergen-specific IgE molecules which attach to the IgE receptor on the surface of mast cell. When that allergen is again encountered specific binding with IgE occurs in such a way that intracellular processes occur resulting in the degranulation of the mast cell and release of numerous mediators. It should be noted that many allergens (including those from pollens and insects) contain proteases which can interrupt the tight junctions and thereby allow allergens to pass through the airway cellular barrier and encounter mast cells and other cells of the innate immune system. Expression of E-cadherin is decreased in the epithelium of asthmatics [18].

Eosinophils play a key role in type 2-high asthma by their pro-inflammatory and immunomodulating functions in the airways. Chemokines such as eotaxins, RANTES and PGD2 attract eosinophils from the bone marrow to the airway within 8–24 hour by binding to receptors CCR3, CCR1 and DP2. Activation occurs with binding of cytokines such as interleukins IL-3 and IL-5 to their corresponding receptors on the eosinophil cell surface, allowing for their presence for 3–8 days. Several features of asthma are a result of their activity. Release of IL-13 and IL-4 causes an upregulation of MUC5AC production and subsequent mucus hyperproduction. Eosinophil extracellular traps (EES) which are extracellular DNA fibers resulting from cellular cytolysis result in increased tenacity of the mucus and correlate with the production of Charcot-Leyden crystals and galectin-10 found in the airways of asthmatic patients. Degranulation of eosinophils releases numerous cytotoxic factors including major binding protein (MBP), eosinophil peroxidase (EPO), eosinophilic cationic protein (ECP), and eosinophil-derived neurotoxin (EDN). These result in epithelial cell damage and can be seen in mucus-epithelial cellular debris and plugs in the asthmatic airway. Other mediators released by the eosinophil include fibrogenic factors such as transforming growth factor-beta (TGF-β) which result in smooth muscle thickening (indicating airway remodeling), goblet cell metaplasia and extracellular matrix protein deposition. Finally, EDN can damage airway nerve fibers and may contribute to AHR. Therefore, pro-inflammatory cytokines such as T2 cytokines (IL-4, IL-5, IL-9, IL-13, IL-25) and chemokines all contribute to the persistence of airway inflammation in type 2-high asthma.

Damage to the epithelium in allergic asthma offers a common pathologic mechanism in other endotypes of ashma as shown in **Figure 2**. Release of proinflammatory cytokines (alarmins) via the nuclear factor-κ B (NF-κB) transcriptional process by the binding of the inhaled allergen to epithelial cell receptors can occur by other receptors or damages to AECs themselves. There is the subsequent infiltration of the airway with eosinophils and the release of their mediators enhance the allergic inflammatory cascade by damaging AECs resulting in further release of alarmins. Instead of an eosinophilic response neutrophils can be seen upon release of their specific chemotactic factors (such as IL-8 and LTB4), from which similar damage to AEC with their phagocytic activity, protease release and apoptosis. This vicious cycle of epithelial damage and inflammation can also occur with various pollutants and irritants in the inhaled air as well as direct viral invasion by respiratory viruses. Increased AHR may be the result of exposed nerve fibers as well as other neuroimmune pathways causing neurogenic inflammation [9]. However exploration of these other inflammatory processes in the airway is beyond this paper's discussion.

Several components of air pollution such as ozone (O_3), sulfur dioxide (SO_2), nitrogen dioxide (NO_2), particulate matter (PM) (especially those less than 2.5 μm or PM2.5), and diesel exhaust particles (DEP) have been shown to be especially damaging to the epithelium and exposure correlates with the clinical development and exacerbation of pediatric asthma [19, 20]. There are several anatomic and biological reasons why infants and children are more susceptible to the effects of toxins in the inhaled air. They have a faster respiratory rate resulting in more exposure and a greater surface area per weight ratio leading to increased deposition. Additionally, since they typically breathe through their nose larger particles in the air avoid the nasal filtration system and are able to pass into the lower respiratory tract. Finally, they often play outside with more exposure to outside particles and especially those heavier ones that are closer to the ground. PM can originate from many sources, including vehicle exhaust, burning of incense and other materials both indoors (e.g., wood-burning stoves) and outdoors (e.g., wildfires), smoking, cooking food (e.g., outside barbeques), sanitary and hygienic sprays, clothing residues, hair or fur from domestic animals and vacuum cleaning. Both type 2 and non-type 2 inflammatory responses can result when air containing these irritants is inhaled. Air pollutants (especially PM2.5) induce epithelial permeability by decreasing the expression of cadherin, catenin, occluding and ZO-1 in airway epithelium thereby allowing for entry of various allergens [21, 22] and subsequent allergic or type 2-high reaction with eosinophilic infiltration. There is the increased secretion of alarmins (IL-25, IL-33, and TSLP) as well as IL-4, IL-5, and IL-13 in subjects exposed to various pollutants. They can also induce secretion of mucus (MUC5AC and MUC5B) as well as causing mucociliary dysfunction by direct effects on cilia activity. Finally, some components can introduce oxidative stress in the cell with the production of reactive oxygen species (ROS) with lipid peroxidation and decreased antioxidant capacity. These all can result the release of IL-8 by AECs leading to neutrophilic involvement and non-type 2 allergic mechanisms such as Th17 pathways and IL-17. Indeed, increased IL-8 from AEC obtained from allergic asthma patients than healthy subjects have been observed. Since non-type 2 high (allergic) asthma is uncommon in children it will not be discussed in this chapter. However, it should be noted that such irritants in the air can trigger both types of inflammatory responses under certain circumstances and enhance the allergic or IgE-mediated mechanism. Interventions to reduce exposure to any of these factors in the air to prevent or lessen the development of asthma will be difficult due to the numerous components present. Limiting exposure to passive smoke is a more possible effort but whether it will decrease the development of asthma remains to be seen [23]. However, lessening their exposure will at least decrease the precipitation of asthmatic attacks and has been reviewed by many studies [24].

Infections by respiratory viruses (especially respiratory syncytial virus or RSV) in children are common and their causative role in asthma still controversial [25–27]. Questions have been raised regarding studies indicating severe or recurrent RSV-associated bronchiolitis during infancy results in an increased risk for both asthma and allergic sensitization [28]. On the other hand infection of the lower respiratory tract by rhinovirus (RV) during the first 3 years of life also appears to increase the risk of asthma by the age of six up to 40-fold [14]. Repeated infections causing asthma symptoms induce AHR in children with atopy. *In vitro* studies with AECs from asthmatics demonstrated that viral infection resulted in typical histological changes with mucus hypersecretion, goblet cell hyperplasia and ASM hypertrophy. There was increased expression of pro-inflammatory genes INF-γ, IL-12 and IL-8 [29].

RV specifically binds to intercellular adhesion molecule 1 (ICAM) on the AEC apical surface to enter the cell. Other receptors include the cadherin-related family member 3 (CDHR3) and low-density lipoprotein receptor (LDL-R). Viral replication is completed with the destruction of the AEC and release of more viral particles. However, whether respiratory viruses can also result in permanent and continued expression of T2 transcriptional and translational processes observed in asthma is not known. Part of the problem is that the underlying mechanisms causing development of asthma may also result in the child and its AECs becoming more susceptible to recurrent or severe respiratory viral infections. These factors include genetic factors (such as atopy), other environmental insults (such as air pollution or cigarette smoke), hormonal imbalances, and nutrition. The infection is usually limited since the body's immune system controls the extent and duration of infection. Virus components result in TLR activation leading to the release of numerous mediators (interferon, defensins, TNF-α, IL-12, IL-6 and chemokine) and in antigen-presenting cell (such as dendritic cell) stimulation of T cell activation. Subsequent immune cell cytotoxicity of infected AECs also contributes to the breakdown of the cellular barrier. Additionally, respiratory viruses can also result in dysfunction of the tight junctions and actin cytoskeleton structures [1]. This disruption of barrier function of the epithelium can result in allergen entry and exposure to mast cells, Th2 cells and dendritic cells; thereby continuing the chronic allergic inflammatory state [30]. It may also explain the occurrence of more serious pathogen infections following viral infections and their role in increasing the risk for asthma. However, asthma symptoms do occur as shown in **Figure 2**. Those children in whom allergic sensitization do not occur may comprise those children who have asthma for a couple of years (also called preschool wheezing) but "outgrow" by adulthood. Novel attempts to prevent the development of allergies or subsequent bacterial infection both of which appear to increase their risk for asthma are in progress [31, 32] since the use of inhaled corticosteroids have not prevented the development of eosinophilic infiltration and continued pulmonary disease. There is increasing evidence that eosinophils have antiviral activities and so the use of biologics such as anti-IL-5 monoclonal antibodies in this population is of interest [33] but needs to be balanced with the possible increased risk of infection [34]. Since airway remodeling already appears between the ages of 1 and 3 years of age before the presence of allergic inflammation an important role for the airway epithelium is suggested and underlies the contributions of genetic predisposition and responses to other environmental exposures.

4. Bronchopulmonary dysplasia (BPD)

BPD was first described in 1967 as a fibrocystic lung disease seen radiologically in premature infants requiring intensive mechanical ventilator support and high concentrations of oxygen during the management of their respiratory distress syndrome (RDS). Despite advances in treatment such as surfactant replacement and antenatal corticosteroid therapy there continued to be a patient population from neonatal intensive care units (NICU) who have long-term respiratory disease throughout childhood and into adulthood as well as significant neurodevelopmental disabilities [35]. Although the traditional definition of BPD continues to be those infants requiring respiratory support at 36 weeks post menstrual age, there is no good delineation of phenotypes predictive of subsequent lung disease. Additionally, there may be factors outside the NICU which can result in chronic disease, termed post-prematurity respiratory disease (PPRD) or neonatal chronic lung disease [36]. Identification of these risk factors include those previously known for BPD such as demographic characteristics (low gestational age, low birth weight, male sex), duration of intensive mechanical ventilation (IMV), and early exposure to inflammation (chorioamnionitis, elevated C-reactive protein, presence of gram-negative bacteria or Ureaplasma organisms). Clinically, the decreasing pulmonary function seen in adolescents and young adults with a history of either BPD or extreme prematurity suggests that PPRD may be a precursor to continued chronic lung disease [33].

The risk factors of intrauterine growth restriction or retardation (IUGR) causing low gestational age and low birth weight in a premature birth will obviously result in a small and underdeveloped lung. Exogenous surfactant has been given to premature infants whose alveolar sacs have remained collapsed due to interruption of the normal maturation of AEC to pneumocytes and lack of surfactant production by Clara and AT-2 cells. Administration results in less energy by the body or mechanical ventilation to expand the sacs and increase gas exchange. However, the use of exogenous surfactant have not decreased the incidence of BPD despite different ways of administering it [37, 38].

Surfactant consists of four proteins, two highly hydrophobic (SP-B and SP-C) and two hydrophilic (SP-A and SP-D), and are assembled into lamellar bodies with phospholipid components. Alveolar decreased surface tension is the result of SP-B and SP-C. SP-A and SP-D as members of a family of anti-microbial proteins called as collectins bind to carbohydrate molecules on the surface of different microorganisms. Several outcomes can result: first, the binding promotes bacterial phagocytosis by neutrophils or macrophages (opsonin activity). Second, the binding to viral-induced molecules on the surface of viral-infected cells such as AEC promotes cell killing by cytotoxic immune cells such natural killer (NK) lymphocytes. Third, direct interaction with various respiratory viruses can result in decreased viral entry and replication within the respiratory tract. Other interactions can result in the killing of other pathogens [39]. They also have a pro-inflammatory role by triggering the release of inflammatory mediators (such as IFN) by binding to AEC and cells of the innate immune systems (such as alveolar macrophages, monocytes, neutrophils). Conversely, they may bind directly to inflammatory mediators to limit cytotoxicity and airway inflammation [40]. Dendritic cell maturation and IL-8 release can be decreased by SP-A. Allergen-induced lymphocyte proliferation and Th-2 cytokine production was inhibited by SP-A and SP-D [41]. Binding of SP to lipopolysaccharide (LPS) decreases LPS-induced inflammation. Therefore, it is uncertain as to whether inflammation will be decreased or enhanced by its administration due to its immunomodulating effects [42]. This may be one reason there has not been a decrease in BPD despite its clinical usage.

Although the administration of surfactant and major treatment advances employing "gentile ventilation" (i.e., using less pressures and volumes in IMV and weaning off supplemental oxygen as soon as possible) the incidence of BPD has not changed. This is because large preterm infants rarely develop BPD but now it occurs in infants weighing less than 1 kg. There has been a change in the lung pathology into what is termed "new" BPD as seen in **Figure 3**. Specifically, there is reduced formation of capillaries (dysmorphic vasculature), mild airway smooth muscle thickening with subsequent alveolar wall thickening, inflammatory cell infiltration with increased alveolar and bronchial cell apoptosis and mild fibrosis, and a combination of both air space enlargement (hyperinflation) and atelectasis. Many aspects of the "new" pathology have been compared to ventilator-induced lung injury (VILI) or acute lung

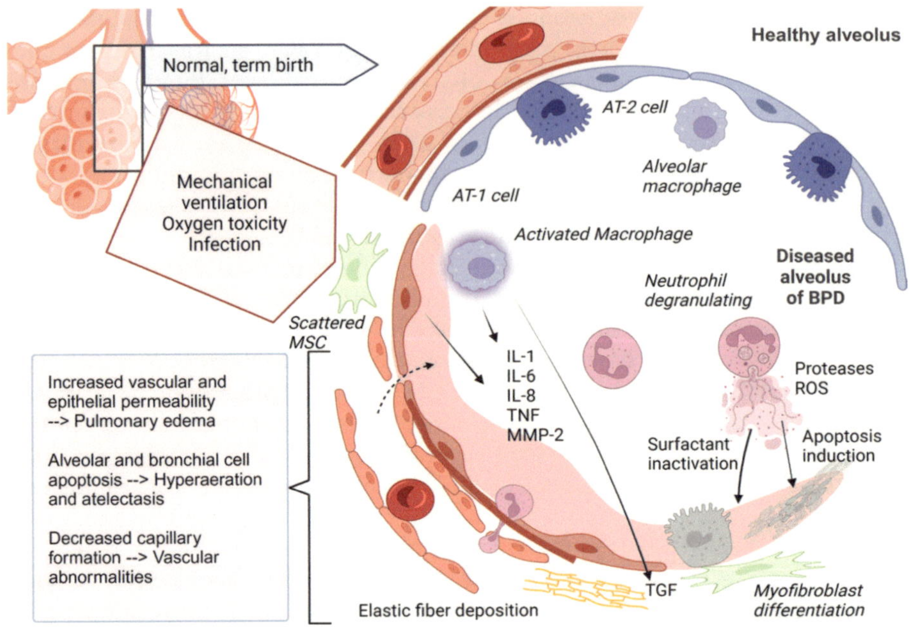

Figure 3.
The inflammatory response in the immature lung as key event leading to bronchopulmonary dysplasia. In a normal, term birth the alveolar airspace is lined with AEC in the form of alveolar type 1 (AT-1) which are flattened to enhance gas exchange between air and blood vessel and alveolar type 2 (AT-2). The cuboidal shaped AT-2 cells produce a thin layer of surfactant, which decreases surface tension, allowing the alveoli to expand with minimal pressure. The alveolar macrophage functions to provide immune protection in the airspace. In a premature birth, mechanical ventilation, oxygen supply and infections induce release of inflammatory mediators by AEC and activated macrophages. The resulting neutrophilic infiltration contributes to the inflammatory response and also results in release of proteases and reactive oxygen species (ROS), disrupting AEC which releases more pro-inflammatory cytokines. This inflammatory overweight disrupts the balanced network of growth signal pathways, affecting the airway epithelium, mesenchyme and vascular endothelium and leading to characteristic features in the lung shown in the box of pulmonary edema, alveolar hyperaeration with atelectasis and vascular abnormalities. Created with BioRender.com.

injury (ALI) with contributions from barotrauma (injury from excessive airway pressure), volutrauma (injury caused by excessive tidal volume), atelectrauma (injury due to repetitive opening and closing of alveoli), as well as oxygen toxicity. Inflammatory mediators (such as IL-1β, IL-6, IL-8, TNF-α and macrophage inflammatory protein-2 (MMP-2)) are seen in tracheal aspirates, BAL, tissue samples and/or blood of BPD patients. Elevated amniotic fluid levels of these cytokines have also been found in mothers whose infants have BPD [43]. Similar pro-inflammatory cytokines have been seen in ventilated animal models (including rats, lambs, and baboons) [44].

Although there has been controversy over the various modes of ventilation and the role of oxygen toxicity, the end result is an accumulation of inflammatory cells and cytokines in the lungs, promoting excessive immune system activation with increased pro-inflammatory cytokines produced (as shown in **Figure 3**). Ventilator induced pressure and volume changes in the lung can trigger inflammatory responses by involving various ionic pore-forming channels with proteins such as Piezo (Piezo 1 and 2) [45] and transient receptor potential vanilloid-type 4 (TRPV4), [46] which respond to mechanical stimuli that stretch or indent the cell membrane of AECs via calcium-dependent mechanisms and a series of intracellular signaling cascades. Pharmacological inhibition of these channels and mouse models deficient in their

DOI: http://dx.doi.org/10.5772/intechopen.1007459

expression resulted in less ALI toward various insults. TRPV4 also appears to be an important regulator of innate hose defense responses such as regulating the response of phagocytic cells (neutrophils and macrophages) to ALI and bacterial clearance in infections. Piezo plays a role both in surfactant production by and also apoptosis of ATII cells. Therefore, in ALI recurring mechanical forces such as those occurring during IMV may involve these mechanosensing proteins regulating both pro- and anti-inflammatory effects and having both beneficial effects in terms of host defense and resolution from lung injury. Another possible mechanism involves the proteoglycans (PG) present in the extracellular matrix (ECM) and in the basement membrane which may "sense" mechanical forces. "One proposed general mechanism … involves the deformation of the long, linear GAG [glycosaminoglycan] chains that are attached to the core protein of the PG. When the ECM experiences mechanical stress from compression, stretch, or fluid flow, the GAG chains can become either compressed or stretched, leading to changes in the PG core protein. These changes in conformation can activate intracellular signaling pathways" [47] similar to those activated by the ion-channel mechanosensory proteins. Thus, TRPV4 activation can result in integrin signaling causing cytoskeletal reorientation, intracellular messengers such as lipid metabolites and kinases. The net effect of disruption of the ECM is further interference of its interactions with other cells (such as mesenchymal cells) in proper morphogenesis and maturation of alveoli structure. The resultant dysregulated collagen deposition and disturbed elastin and laminin fiber organization are typical features of the BPD lung. Airway inflammation was lessened by using various TRPV4 antagonists in allergen challenged pre-sensitized animals or genetic knockout mice [48]. However, thus far, there has been no attempt in using TRPV4 antagonists and Piezo ligands in BPD.

In addition to the pro-inflammatory effects of IMV, supplemental oxygen or hyperoxia exposure can also independently damage the immature lungs, mainly due to the immaturity of its antioxidative systems and initial effects on the alveolar macrophage. There are lower levels of antioxidant enzymes such as superoxide dismutase (SOD) and glutathione (GSH) as well as nonenzyme antioxidants such as vitamins A, C and E in premature infants as compared to term neonates [49]. Excessive levels of oxidative products have also been found in tracheal aspirates of BPD infants [50]. Exposure to high concentrations of oxygen results in decrease production of IL-1β, IL-6 and TNF-α but an increase in IL-8 [51]. There is continued activation of macrophages due to a lack of surfactant proteins, which can downregulate the activity of alveolar macrophages. Potent oxidants (such as hypochlorous acid) and proteases (such as elastase and metalloproteinases) from the infiltrated neutrophils damage the AEC, especially AT-2 and Clara cells. This further decreases the presence of surfactant, which also suffers from direct inactivation by reactive oxidant species (ROS). Injured AECs further release mediators such as IL-8 drawing more neutrophils and continues the release of oxidants. However, the overall contribution of hyperoxia to inflammation appears to be moderate and so other animal models have combined oxygen exposure to infection by adding LPS which did result in dose-dependent inflammatory reactions and even systemic inflammatory response (depending upon the species, strain and LPS dosage). This may explain why treatment with supplemental antioxidants such as vitamins A and E although helpful has not significantly decreased the overall incidence of BPD.

There is much clinical and experimental evidence that varying types of prenatal and antenatal infections play a role in inducing inflammation. Associations between the development of BPD have been seen not only in various gram negative bacteria with LPS but also in viral infection [52] and presence of *Ureaplasma urealyticum* [53]. Therefore, inflammation whether by infectious process and "sterile" mechanisms appear to result in the pathology seen in BPD. BPD is unique in that the lung is immature and therefore there is a need for alveolar and vascular growth to develop normally outside of the maternal environment. The process of lung morphogenesis depends upon multiple signaling pathways controlling cellular proliferation, survival and differentiation and coordinating with those signal cascades regulating vascular development. Therefore there must be a close relationship between blood vessels and airways with coordinated interplay of growth factors and angiogenetic transcriptional pathways such as hypoxic inducible factor (HIF), NF-κB, nitric oxide and nitric oxide synthase (NOS) among others. These are balanced with anti-angiogenic molecules such as angiopoietin 1 and endostatin [54]. AT-2 pneumocytes produce vascular endothelial growth factor (VEGF) which promotes angiogenesis suggesting that treatment with VEGF may be beneficial. Decreased VEGF levels have been observed in premature birth, especially those who later develop BPD [55]. Since the main stimuli for VEGF production by AEC is hypoxia, treatment with supplemental oxygen can actually decrease its production. Decreased VEGF production results in increased alveolar and bronchial cell apoptosis, air space enlargement and changes in elastin. This aspect has been termed the "vascular hypothesis" of BPD and suggests the potential use of pro-angiogenetic agents in BPD. Additionally, endostatin opposes VEGF and the coordinate activities of both cytokines guide the developing avasculature by myofibroblast and mesenchymal stem cell (MSC) differentiation. Similarly, Angiopoietin-1 (Ang-1) stabilizes new blood vessels and angiopoietin-2 (Ang-2) opposes Ang-1 activity by impairing vessel stability resulting in excessive vessel "sprouting". Elevated levels of endostatin and reduced ratio of Ang-1 to Ang-2 have been seen in lung fluid from BPD patients [56]. MSC differentiation and activity is affected by the excessive activity in the TGF-β and NFκB pathways. Therefore, the excessive proinflammatory response appears to result in suppression of vascular growth promoting cytokines. The inflammatory cytokines is appears early after birth and before the deterioration of lung function [57]. As noted above, there are effects on the epithelial cell structure and function at both the bronchiolar and alveolar levels.

Another characteristic of BPD is the presence of pulmonary edema from increased permeability, resulting in a clinical management challenges in fluid management and adequate nutrition. However, the mechanism of the increased vascular permeability has not been clearly delineated. One possibility is the immaturity of the tight junction formation between cells in both the airway epithelium and vascular endothelium due to the premature birth. Defective expression of tight junction proteins such as claudins (especially claudin-4 and claudin 18), occludin and zonal occludens-1 (ZO-1) has also been found with exposure to hyperoxia in both *in vitro* models. Further support is suggested by the lack of claudin-28 resulting in histophathology similar to human BPD in knock-out mice with barrier dysfunction and impaired alveolar development [38]. Additionally, the amount of desmosome proteins are less in BPD infants. Diuretic therapy has been used but long term use has been complicated by electrolyte losses causing metabolic bone disease, nephrocalcinosis and growth failure and controversy over its efficacy [58]. However, another possible mode of action of furosemide in BPD is its anti-antiflammatory effect [59]. There has been some suggestion that diuretics may additionally have immunomodulating effect [60].

In summary, a key role is seen for the epithelium in BPD and the various factors which has been associated with its development. Mechanical ventilation, oxygen stress and infection can all trigger an inflammatory reaction initially characterized by involvement of alveolar macrophages and neutrophils. Their activity results in epithelial cell involvement and the resulting proinflammatory loop between macrophages, neutrophils and epithelial cells damages the developing vascular and respiratory components. The increased predilection for female sex may be explained by the increased immune activity of neutrophils (and possibly macrophages). However, there is currently no reliable biomarker that reliably predicts which neonates will develop BPD as evidenced by distorted alveolarization and impaired vasculogenesis; or can be used to monitor its progression [35].

5. Cystic fibrosis (CF)

Cystic fibrosis (CF) is a genetic disorder due to a defective expression of the cystic fibrosis transmembrane conductance regulator (CFTR) gene primarily affecting the respiratory and gastrointestinal systems. Severe mutations result in symptoms starting in infancy with steatorrhea, poor weight gain and respiratory symptoms of coughing and/or wheezing. Chronic respiratory bacterial infections occur with progressive loss of lung function. Therefore, it is not surprising that chronic inflammation has been long-recognized as an important component of the immunopathogenesis of CF [61] and it appears a dominant T2 response has been identified [62]. At birth the histology of the lungs are normal but with increasing age an inflammatory response is seen with the occurrence of mucus plugs in the airways corresponding to elevated levels of IL-8 and neutrophil elasase in BAL or tracheal washings and blood. It had been assumed that infectious pathogens were responsible, initially *Staphylococcus aureus* and then *Pseudomonas aeruginosa* [63]. Microbial organisms (including other pathogens such as fungi) become trapped by the thick tenacious mucus produced as a result of the CFTR genetic defect. Impaired mechanical eradication results from the inability of the mucociliary clearance (MCC) mechanism to remove the thick mucus-bacteria. When about 75% of the CFTR activity is absent in the airway, the mucus is thick enough to result in decreased MCC [64].

Function of CFTR is to regulate chloride transport across the cellular membrane of many cell types, but especially epithelial cells in both respiratory and gastrointestinal systems. With decreasing CFTR activity in *the airway* epithelial cells there is an increase in intracellular Cl^- and HCO_3^+ and increase absorption of Na^+ (via a functioning ENaC channel) and water from the luminal surface resulting in a dehydrated and acidic ASL in the airway (see **Figure 4**). Dysfunctional CFTR results in defective antimicrobial killing prolonging the persistence of bacteria and three different hypothesis have been proposed for the exact mechanism [65]. Some have speculated that there is defective killing of bacteria by the neutrophils due to the high salt concentration of the luminal mucus, the high salt hypothesis. However, there have been conflicting reports measuring the salt ion concentration in the ASL. The acidic hypothesis states that the decreased bacterial killing is due to the reduction of antimicrobial activities of neutrophic enzymes such as lysozyme and lactoferrin, as well as defensin-3 in the acidic pH ASL environment. Although there has been much experimental support in *in vitro* systems, direct measurements of ASL pH in animals reveal confusing results, indicating involvement of many other factors (such as age and other mechanisms) [44]. These two mechanisms indicate defective phagocytic processes where the engulfed bacteria is not able to be killed within the phagosome. Finally, the ASL water content is decreased, resulting in a dehydrated mucus layer. The overall net effect of CFTR dysfunction is an abnormal ASL with chronic infection

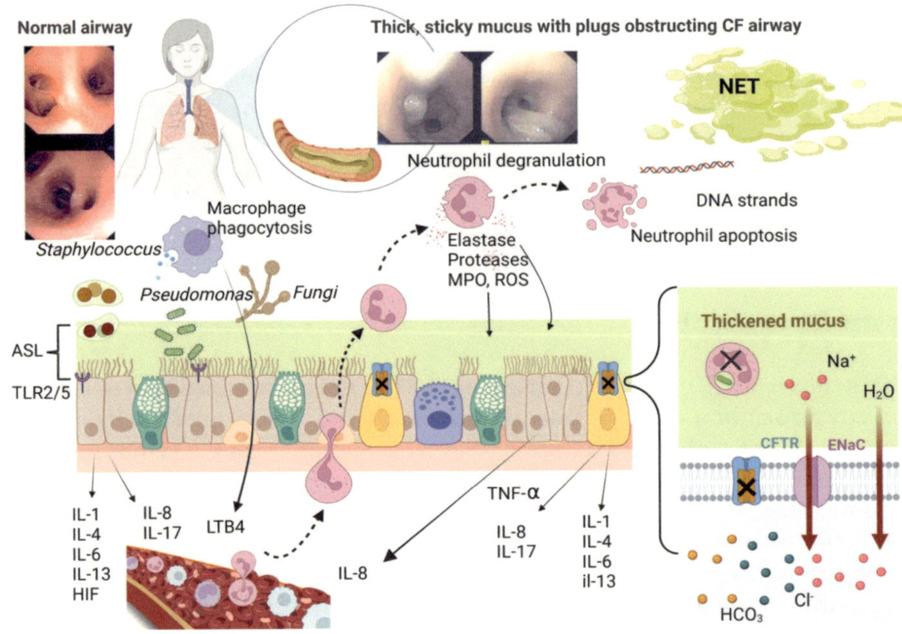

Figure 4.
Immunopathologic mechanisms in CF airway with involvement airway epithelial cells (AECs). A typical CF patient has excessive mucus resulting in mucus obstruction and airway narrowing as shown by the inserted pictures by bronchoscopy of normal and CF airways. The basis for thickened mucus is shown in the close-up depiction of the interface between the cell membrane and air-space fluid (ASL). Defective CFTR protein results in an accumulation of intracellular Cl^- and HCO_3^+ ions . There is also increased activity of the ENaC transporting Na^+ ions from the ASL to inside the cell, which draws water inside the cell. (Although not shown, defective CFTR is present in all the cells.) The net result is a dehydrated acidic ASL and a thick, sticky mucus which result in AECs releasing inflammatory cytokines, especially IL-8, drawing neutrophils into the airway from the blood vessel. Neutrophilic infiltration can also be the result of the binding of bacteria and other pathogens such as fungi to AEC TLR receptors and by the release of other chemokines such as leukotriene LTB4 by activated macrophages with the presence of various pathogens. The overall result is an intense neutrophilic presence which further damages the airway by the release of proteolytic enzymes such as myeloperoxidase oxidase (MPO) and reactive oxygen species (ROS). Additionally, the neutrophils undergo apoptosis and its chromatin/DNA then forms a neutrohilc extracellular net (NET), further increasing ASL viscosity. Mucus plugs result subsequent hypoxia under the ASL inducing the hypoxia inducible factor (HIF) pathway leading to more IL-8 release and the inflammatory cycle continues with IL-17 and TNF-α stimulating goblet cell mucus production. Created with BioRender.com.

resulting in mucus plugs and continuing inflammation despite the use of highly effective CFTR modulator therapy [66].

AECs responds to the presence of bacteria by releasing a set of pro-inflammatory cytokines including IL-4, IL-1β, IL-13, IL-8, IL-17 and TNF-α after components of the bacteria, mainly lipopolysaccharide (LPS), bind to TLR2/5 receptors. All of these have been found to be increased in sputum and BAL from CF patients [43]. Since some of these cytokines are relevant to asthma and allergic processes it should not be surprisingly that a significant number of patients with CF also have these disorders as well. However, the persistent production and release of IL-8 and IL-17 from continued presence of bacteria results in increasing neutrophilic inflammation in the CF airway. It should be noted that several of the inflammatory cytokines also induce HCO_3^+ secretion across the airway epithelia by increasing the activities of CFTR and pendrin channels. However, since CF has defective CFTR the ASL remains acidic making bacterial eradication difficult.

In addition the inability of the neutrophils to kill bacteria, they themselves become a source of proteases, especially elastase, which could be detrimental to the epithelium [67]. Elastase has been correlated with the severity of CF lung disease and has served as a marker for the effectiveness of any therapeutic modalities. Its expression is further increased by the proinflammatory cytokine TNF-α. Although there is no evidence that elastase is directly cytotoxic to AEC, it can damage the AJ protein E-cadherin and thereby increase the epithelium permeability. It also increases MUC5AC and so contributes to the mucus obstruction of airways. Other cellular contents of the neutrophils such as myeloperoxidase (MPO) are also released in the ASL resulting in an increase in its pro-oxidant environment and contributing to damage to AEC, which further releases more IL-8 and IL-17. However, there are other mediators such as matrix metalloproteinase (MMP)-8 which are anti-inflammatory. Other neutrophilic chemoattractants such as leukotriene B4 (LTB4) are produced by alveolar macrophages as a response to the presence of bacteria. Increased levels of LTB4 and the complement system-derived C5a have also been found in various CF respiratory fluids [68]. The net effect is the development of neutrophil extracellular trap (NET). The neutrophils undergo a process similar to apoptosis termed NETosis, in which there is release of chromatin as well as their granules. This innate host defense is an attempt to block microbial organisms from spreading and facilitate their killing and phagocytosis and is especially common in fungal infections, such as *Aspergillus fumigatus* which is common in CF. Components of the neutrophils such as the actin and DNA surround the organisms to form an enclosed compartment. However, the release DNA contributes to the increased thickness and viscosity of the ASL which the MCC is unable to clear (see **Figure 4**). There is actually very little intact mucin present but instead increased amounts of large macromolecules including DNA, filamentous actin, lipids, and proteoglycans with is responsible for the increased thickness of CF sputum [69]. Acknowledging its importance there has been successful treatment with the enzyme DNase which breaks down DNA strands [70].

There is evidence that airway inflammation is present without evidence of infection [48]. In studies of infants before bacterial presence as detected by its DNA by polymerase chain reaction (PCR) inflammatory cytokines such as IL-8 and elastase indicating the presence of neutrophils are detected in BAL or tracheal washings. Additionally, CF infants who die within weeks or months after birth already show airway lumen filled and plugged by mucus plugs comprising of neutrophilic debris. Three possible mechanisms for this "sterile" airway inflammation have been proposed. One is the presence of altered ASL. The cells which have predominant CFTR expression are the ionocytes, goblet cells and secretory cells in the submuosal glands. Altered CFTR protein decreases the hydration and possibly the pH of ASL as noted above. However, although measurements of pH in ASL in nasal secretions were lower in CF infants at birth compared to normal no differences were seen in repeat measurements at 3 months of age [63]. There is also Na^+ hyperabsorption due to excessive activity of ENaC resulting in low ASL volume with cilia deformities and also decreased MCC. Some support has been found in transgenic mice overexpressing ENaC and resulting in CF-like lung inflammation and disease. However, its contribution may be minimal since clinical treatment with hypertonic solutions was only moderate and short-term.

The other possible mechanism for sterile inflammation by neutrophils is the localized area of hypoxia caused by mucus plugs and increased ENaC activity [71]. The thick stagnant ASL creates a steep oxygen gradient exposing the underlying AECs to hypoxic conditions. Indeed, measurements in CF patients indicate the presence of oxygen at less than 10 mmHg (which corresponds to less than 1–2% O_2 air-content) in certain areas of the lungs [72]. The hypoxia results in the production of hypoxic inducible factor (HIF) which then promotes the release of inflammatory factors, IL-4, IL-5, IL-13, and TNF-β. Additionally, we have found that IL-8 is also produced by AEC line lines exposed to anoxic conditions [73]. Finally, HIF also induces TH17 cell differentiation [74].

Finally, there may be intrinsic defects within the AEC itself in terms of IL-8 production at the genetic level. Specifically, differences in the histone acetyltransferase (HAT)/HDAC balance, histone and DNA methylation, and miRNA-dependent post-transcriptional regulation in AEC from CF and normal subjects have been found [48]. Whether these alterations in signal transduction are clinically relevant is not known.

In the CF airway the major problem is the clearance of mucus in the ASL. The thickened mucus is due to several factors. There is the genetic defect in AEC transport of ions between the cell membrane and airway lumen. Inflammatory processes by activation of AEC either by the abnormal acidic mucus or localized hypoxia triggers an inflammatory response resulting in neutrophilic infiltration, which is furthered enhanced by antimicrobial immune defense toward specific infectious pathogens which appears to specifically colonize the CF patient. The resultant NET contributes to the tenacity of the mucus layer with resultant mucus plugs and the clinical sequalae. Unlike the allergic asthmatic in whom the eosinophil contributes to the airway inflammation s mucus plugs are rarely seen. The MCC is not as compromised and pathogen driven inflammation is not present on a continual basis.

6. Conclusions

The airway epithelium serves as a barrier between the body and external environment with potentially harmful agents such as respiratory pathogens and toxic gases. Protection is provided in several layers. There is a physical barrier of epithelial cells which is supported by a chemical defense in the form of antimicrobial molecules, proinflammatory cytokines and chemotines, and mucus entrapment and elimination through a mucus clearing system. Finally, it comprises an important part of the innate immune system in protecting it against numerous pathogens. This chapter reviews its involvement in the immunopathogenesis of three pediatric respiratory disorders. Understanding its role allows insights into how current treatment modalities are effective and the development of potentially future therapies.

The importance of the AECs in asthma, bronchopulmonary dysplasia (BPD) and cystic fibrois (CF) is shown by its role in regulating lung homeostasis with open airways and adequate gas exchange. Mucus can be the result of stimulation of secretory cells in response to exposure to potentially harmful substances in the inhaled air such as pathogens, allergens or toxins and its effective clearance by the mucociliary clearance. However, excessive amounts can be produced with continued exposure or unusually thick mucus by genetic defects in the cells. These could be from a defective CFTR protein in CF or genetic predispositions in IgE production in allergic asthma. The integrity of the epithelium barrier can also be compromised by procedures needed to support premature infants with intensive mechanical ventilation and high levels of supplemental oxygen in the presence of an underdeveloped lung and vascular structure and immature immune system. These three scenarios precipitate an inflammatory response from the lung innate immune system. In asthma it commonly results in an eosinophilic airway presence whereas in CF neutrophils are present. There is a complex interaction among alveolar macrophages, neutrophils and epithelial cells in BPD that results in increased pro-inflammatory cytokines which is similar to that seen in asthma and CF. Therefore, it is not surprisingly that anti-inflammatory therapies such as corticosteroids have been used in each of these three disorders. Discussion of their specific effects in each disease is beyond the scope of this review. However, understanding of the nature of the specific inflammatory process can allow for more specific targeting of each condition. This may involve using specific stem cells as well as monoclonal antibody-based pharmacologic interventions.

Conflict of interest

The author declares no conflict of interest.

Author details

Terry Chin
University of California, Irvine, Irvine, California, USA

*Address all correspondence to: twchin1224@gmail.com

References

[1] Rezaee F, Georgas SN. Breaking barriers: New insights into airway epithelial barrier function in health and disease. American Journal of Respiratory Cellular and Molecular Biology. 2014;**50**:857-869. DOI: 10.1165/rcmb.2013-0541RT

[2] Davis JD, Wypych TP. Cellular and functional heterogeneity of the airway epithelium. Mucosal: Immunology. 2021;**14**:978-990. DOI: 10.1038/s41385-020-00370-7

[3] Meng X, Cui G, Peng C. Lung development and regeneration: Newly defined cell types and progenitor status. Cell Regeneration. 2023;**12**:5. DOI: 10.1038/s41385-020-00370-7

[4] Thakur A, Mei S, Zhang N, Zhang K, Taslakjian B, Lian J, et al. Pulmonary neuroendocrine cells: Crucial players in respiratory function and airway-nerve communication. Frontiers in Neuroscience. 2024;**18**. DOI: 10.3389/fnins.2024.1438188

[5] Bukowy-Bieryllo Z. Long-term differentiating primary human airway epithelial cell cultures: How far are we? Cell Communication and Signaling. 2021;**19**:63. DOI: 10.1186/s12964-021-00740-z

[6] Chen J, Lai X, Song Y, Su X. Neuroimmune recognition and regulation in the respiratory system. European Respiratory Review. 2024;**33**:240008. DOI: 10.1183/16000617.0008-2024

[7] Lucchini CA, Nin G, Rossi A, Dorward D, Lucas C. Epithelial cells and inflammation in pulmonary wound repair. Cells. 2021;**10**:339. DOI: 10.3390/cells10020339

[8] Lu H, Cao P. Neural mechanisms underlying the coughing reflex. Neuroscience Bulletin. 2023;**39**:1823-1839. DOI: 10.1007/s12264-023-01104-y

[9] Trevizan-Bau P, Mazzone SB. Neuroimmune pathways regulating airway inflammation. Annals of Allergy, Asthma & Immunology. 2023;**131**:550-560. DOI: 10.1016/j.anai.2023.07.020

[10] Man SM, Kanneganti TD. Innate immune sensing of cell death in disease and therapeutics. Nature Cell Biology. 2024;**26**:1420-1433. DOI: 10.1038/s41556-024-01491-y

[11] Global Initiative for Asthma. Global Strategy for Asthma Management and Prevention (2024 update). Available from: www.oinasthma.org [Accessed: September 01, 2024]

[12] Lotvall J, Akdis CA, Bacharier LB, Bjermer L, Casale TV, Custovic A, et al. Asthma endotypes: A new approach to classification of disease within the entities asthma syndrome. Journal of Allergy and Clinical Immunology. 2011;**127**:355-360. DOI: 10.1016/j.jaci.2010.11.037

[13] Conrad LA, Cabana MD, Rastogi D. Defining pediatric asthma: Phenotypes to endotypes and beyond. Pediatric Research. 2021;**90**:45-51. DOI: 10.1038/s41390-020-01231-6

[14] Gauvreau GM, El-Gammal AI, O'Byrne PM. Allergen-induced airway responses. European Respiratory Journal. 2015;**46**:819-831. DOI: 10.1183/13993003.00536-2015

[15] Fauquert J, Alba-Linero C, Testera-Montes A, Bentabol-Ramos GS.

Allergen-specific allergen challenges in airway allergy: Current utilities and future directions. Allergy. 2023;**78**:1794-1809. DOI: 10.1111/all.15731

[16] Molderings GJ, Afrin LB. A survey of the currently known mast cell mediators with potential relevance for therapy of mast cell-induced symptoms. Naunyn-Schmiedeberg's Archives of Pharmacology. 2023;**396**:2881-2891. DOI: 10.1007/s00210-023-02545-y

[17] Bradding P, Porsbjerg C, Cote A, Dahlen S-E, Hallstrand TS, Brightling CE. Airway hyperresonsiveness in asthma: The role of the epithelium. Journal of Allergy and Clinical Immunology. 2024;**153**:1181-1193. DOI: 10.1016/j.jaci.2024.02.011

[18] Russell RJ, Boulet L-P, Brightling CE, Pavord ID, Porsbjerg C, Dorscheid D, et al. The airway epithelium: An orchestrator of inflammation, a key structural barrier and a therapeutic target in severe asthma. European Respiratory Journal. 2024;**63**:2301397. DOI: 10.1183/13993003.01397-2023

[19] Zhou X, Sampath V, Nadeau KC. Effect of air pollution on asthma. Annals of Allergy, Asthma & Immunology. 2024;**132**:426-432. DOI: 10.1016/j.anai.2024.01.017

[20] Sun BZ, Gaffin JM. Recent insights into the environmental determinants of childhood asthma. Current Allergy and Asthma Reports. 2024;**24**:253-260. DOI: 10.1007/s11882-024-01140-2

[21] Aghapour M, Ubags NK, Bruder D, Hiemstra PS, Sidhaye V, Rezaee F, et al. Role of air pollutants in airway epithelial barrier dysfunctin in asthma and COPD. European Respiratory Research. 2022;**31**:210112. DOI: 10.1183/160000617.0112-2021

[22] Kayalar O, Rajabi H, Konyalilar N, Mortazavi D, Aksoy GT, Wang J, et al. Impact of particulate air pollution on airway injury and epithelial plasticity; underlying mechanisms. Frontiers in Immunology. 2024;**15**:1324552. DOI: 10.3389/fimmu.2024.1324552

[23] Kaur J, Upendra S, Barde S. "Inhaling hazards, exhaling insights": A systematic review unveiling the silent health impacts of secondhand smoke pollution on children and adolescents. International Journal of Environmental Health Research. 2024:1-25. DOI: 10.1080/09603123.2024.2337837

[24] Wang J, Cortes-Ramirez J, Gan T, Davies JM, Hu W. Effects of climate and environmental factors on childhood and adolescent asthma: A systematic review based on spatial and temporal analysis. Science of the Total Environment. 2024;**951**:e175863. DOI: 10.1016/j.scitotenv.2024.175863

[25] Rosas-Salazar C, Chirkova T, Gebretsadik T, et al. Respiratory syncytial virus infection during infancy and asthma during childhood in the USA (INSPIRE): A population-based, prospective birth cohort study. Lancet. 2023;**401**(10389):1669-1680. DOI: 10.1016/S0140-6736(23)00811-5

[26] Ong S. The search for a connection between RSV and asthma. Nature. 2023;**621**(7980):S64-S65. DOI: 10.1038/d41586-023-02961-3

[27] Su P, Jiang C, Zhang Y. The implications of infection with respiratory syncytial virus in pediatric recurrent wheezing and asthma: Knowledge expanded post-COVID-19 era. European Journal of Clinical Microbiology & Infectious Diseases. 2024;**43**:403-416. DOI: 10.1007/s10096-023-04744-0

[28] Shiroshita A, Gebretsadik T, Wu P, Kubilay NZ, Hartert TV. Association between age of respiratory syncytial virus infection hospitalization and childhood asthma: A systematic review. PLoS One. 2024;**19**:e0296685. DOI: 10.1371/journal.pone.0296685

[29] Berdnikovs S, Newcomb DC, Hartert TV. How early life respiratory viral infections impact airway epithelial development and may lead to asthma. Frontiers in Pediatrics. 2024;**12**:1441293. DOI: 10.3389/fped.2024.1441293

[30] Pace E, DiVincernzo S, Ferraro M, Lanata L, Scagione F. Role of airway epithelium in viral respiratory infections: Can carbocysteine prevent or mitigate them? Immunology. 2024;**172**:329-342. DOI: 10.1111/imm.13762

[31] Saglani S. Preventing progression of preschool wheezing to asthma: Opportunities for intervention. Pediatric Allergy and Immunology. 2024;**35**:e14180. DOI: 10.1111/pai.14180

[32] Papadopoulos NG, Apostolidou E, Milighos M, Kepapadaki. Bacteria and viruses and their role in the preschool wheeze to asthma transition. Pediatric Allergy and Immunology. 2024;**35**:e14098. DOI: 10.1111/pai.14098

[33] Rupani H, Busse WW, Howarth PH, Bardin PG, Adcock IM, Konno S, et al. Therapeutic relevance of eosinophlic inflammation and airway viral interactions in severe asthma. Allergy. 2024:16242. DOI: 10.1111/all.16242

[34] Giossi R, Pani A, Schroeder J, Scaglione F. Exploring the risk of infection events in patients with asthma receiving anti-IL-5 monoclonal antibodies: A rapid systematic review and a metaanalysis. Heliyon. 2024;**10**:e23725. DOI: 10.1016/j.heliyon.2023.e23725

[35] Wozniak PS, Makhoul L, Botros MM. Bronchopulmonary dysplasia in adults: Exploring pathogenesis and phenotype. Pediatric Pulmonology. 2024;**59**:540-551

[36] Gilfillan MA, Mejia MJ, Bhandari V. Prevalence, prevention and management of bronchopulmonary dysplaia. Research and Reports in Neonatology. 2024;**14**:1-33. DOI: 10.2147/RRN.S405985

[37] Bonadies L, Zaramella P, Porzionato A, Perilongo G, Muraca M, Baraldi E. Present and future of bronchopulmonary dysplasia. Journal of Clinical Medicine. 2020;**9**:1539. DOI: 10.3390/jcm9051539

[38] El-Atawi K, Abdul Wahab M, Alallah J, et al. Beyond Bronchopulmonary dysplasia: A comprehensive review of chronic lung diseases in neonates. Cureus. 2024;**16**(7):e64804. DOI: 10.7759/cureus.64804

[39] Zhou C, Wong Y. Structure–activity relationship of cationic surfactants as antimicrobial agents. Current Opinion in Colloid & Interface Science. 2020;**45**:28-43. DOI: 10.1016/j.cocis.2019.11.009

[40] Isasi-Campillo M, Lasada-Oliva P, Perez-Gil J, Olmeda B, Garcia-Ortega L. Pulmonary surfactant-derived antiviral actions at the resiratory surface. Current Opinion in Colloid & Interface Science. 2023;**66**:101711. DOI: 10.1016/j.cocis.2023.101711

[41] Watson A, Madsen J, Clark H. SP-A and SP-D: Dual functioning immune molecules with antiviral and immunomodulatory properties. Frontiers in Immunology. 2021:622598. DOI: 10.3389/fimmu.2020.622598

[42] Dong S, Pang H, Li F, Hua M, Liang M, Song C. Immunoregulatory function of SP-A. Molecular

Immunology. 2024;**166**:58-64. DOI: 10.1016/j.molimm.2024.01.005

[43] Mizikcik I, Thebald B. Perinatal origins of bronchopulmonary dysplasia: Deciphering normal and impaired lung development cell by cell. Molecular and Cellular Pediatrics. 2023;**10**:4. DOI: 10.1186/s40348-023-00158-2

[44] Dankhara N, Holla I, Ramarao S, Thekkeveedu RK. Bronchopulmonary dysplasia: Pathogenesis and pathophysiology. Journal of Clinical Medicine. 2023;**12**:4207. DOI: 10.3390/jcm12134207

[45] Jairaman A, Prakriya M. Calcium signaling in airway epithelial cells: Current understanding andimplicaions for inflammatory airway disease. Arteriosclerosis, Thrombosis, and Vascular Biology. 2024;**44**:772-783. DOI: 10.1161/atvbaha.123.318339

[46] Michalick L, Kuebler WM. TRPV4—A missing link between mechanosensation and immunity. Fontiers in Immunology. 2020;**11**:413. DOI: 10.3389/fimmu.2020.00413

[47] Farach-Carson MC, Wu D, Franca CM. Proteoglycans in mechanobiology of tissues and organs: Normal functions and mechanopathology. Proteoglycan Research. 2023;**2**:e21. DOI: 10.1002/pgr2.21

[48] Burgess JK, Gosens R. Mechanotransduction and the extracellular matrix: Key drivers of lung pathologies and drug responsiveness. Biochemical Pharmacology. 2024;**228**:116255. DOI: 10.1016/j.bcp.2024.116255

[49] Kimble A, Robbins ME, Perez M. Pathogenesis of bronchopulmonary dysplasia: Role of oxidative stress from 'Omics' studies. Antioxidants. 2022;**11**:2380. DOI: 10.3390/antiox11122380

[50] Wu T-J, Jing X, Teng M, Pritchard KA, Day BW, Naylor S, et al. Role of myeloperoxidase, oxidative stress, and inflammation in bronchopulmonary dysplasia. Antioxidants. 2024;**13**:889. DOI: 10.3390/antiox13080889

[51] Zaloudikova M. Mechanisms and effects of macrophage polarization and its specifics in pulmonary environment. Physiology Research. 2023;**72**(Suppl 2):S137-S156. DOI: 10.33549/physiolres.935058

[52] Guo X, Ma D, Li R, Zhang R, Guo Y, Yu Z, et al. Association between viral infection and bronchopulmonary dysplasia in preterm infants: A systematic review and meta-analysis. European Journal of Pediatrics. 2024:1-17. DOI: 10.1007/s00431-024-05565-9

[53] Chen X, Huang X, Zhou Q, Kang H, Qiu H, Shi L, et al. Association between *Ureaplasma urealyticum* colonization and bronchopulmonary dysplasia in preterm infants: A systematic review and meta-analysis. Frontiers in Pediatrics. 2024;**12**:1436568. DOI: 10.3389/fped.2024.1436568

[54] Durlak W, Thebaud B. The vascular phenotype of BPD: New basic science insights—New precision medicine approaches. Pediatric Research. 2022. DOI: 10.1038/s41390-022-02428-7

[55] Perrone S, Manti S, Buttarelli L, Petrolini C, Boscarino G, Filonzi L, et al. Vascular endothelial growth factor as molecular target for bronchopulmonary dysplasia prevention in very low birth weight infants. International Journal of Molecular Sciences. 2023;**24**:2729. DOI: 10.3390/ijms24032729

[56] Mathew R. Signaling pathways involved in the development of bronchopulmonary dysplasia and plmonary hypertension. Children. 2002;**7**:100. DOI: 10.3390/children7080100

[57] Holzfurtner L, Shahzad T, Dong Y, Rekers L, Selting A, Staude B, et al. When inflammation meets lung development—An update on the pathogenesis of bronchopulmonary dysplasia. Molecular and Cellular Pediatrics. 2022;**9**:7. DOI: 10.1186/s40348-022-00137-z

[58] Briain EÓ, Byrne AO, Dowling J, Kiernan J, Lynch JC, Alomairi L, et al. Diuretics use in the management of bronchopulmonary dysplasia in preterm infants: A systematic review. Acta Paediatrica. 2024;**113**:394-402. DOI: 10.1111/apa.17093

[59] Yuengsrigul A, Chin TW, Nussbaum E. Immunosuppressive and cytotoxic effects of furosemide on human peripheral blood mononuclear cells. Annals of Allergy, Asthma, & Immunology. 1999;**83**:559-566. DOI: 10.1016/s1081-1206(10)62870-0

[60] Bryniarski P, Nazimek K, Marcinkiewicz J. Immunomodulatory Potential of Diuretics. Biology. 2021;**13**:1315. DOI: 10.3390/biology10121315

[61] Chmiel JF, Berger M, Konstan MW. The role of inflammation in the pathophysiology of CF lung disease. Clinical Reviews in Allergy & Immunology. 2002;**23**:5-27. DOI: 10.1385/CRIAI:23:1:005

[62] Purushothaman AK, Nelson EJR. Role of innate immunity and systemic inflammation in cystic fibrosis disease progression. Heliyon. 2023;**9**:e17553. DOI: 10.1016/j.heliyon.2023.e17553

[63] Sheykhsaran E, Abbasi A, Memar MY, et al. The role of *Staphylococcus aureus* in cystic fibrosis pathogenesis and clinico-microbiological interactions. Diagnostic Microbiology and Infections Disease. 2024;**109**:116294. DOI: 10.1016/j.diagmicrobio.2024.116294

[64] Ahang L, Button B, Gabriel SE, Burkett YY, et al. CFTR delivery to 25% of surface epithelial cells restores normal rates f mucus transport to human cystic fibrosis airway epithelium. PLoS. 2009;**7**:e1000155. DOI: 10.1371/journal.pbio.1000155

[65] Wu M, Chen J-H. CFTR dysfunction leads to defective bacterial eradication on cystic fibrosis airways. Frontiers in Physiology. 2024;**15**:1385661. DOI: 10.3389/fphys.2024.1385661

[66] Rehman T, Welsh MJ. Inflammation as a regulator of the airway surface liquid pH in cystic fibrosis. Cells. 2023;**12**:1104. DOI: 10.3390/cells12081104

[67] Haynes ME, Sullivan DP, Muller WA. Neutrophilic infiltration and function in the pathogenesis of inflammatory airspace disease. American Journal of Pathology. 2024;**194**:628-636. DOI: 10.1016/j.ajpath.2023.12.008

[68] Cabrini G, Rimessi A, Borgatti M, Lamprointi I, Finotti A, Pinton P, et al. Role of cystic fibrosis bronchial epithelium in neutrophil chemotaxis. Frontiers in Immunology. 2020;**11**:143. DOI: 10.3389/fimmu.2020.0143

[69] Voynow JA, Rubin BK. Mucins, mucus, and sputum. Chest. 2009;**135**:505-512. DOI: 10.1378/chest.08-0412

[70] Roesch EA, Rahmaoui A, Lazarus RA, Konstan MW. The continuing need for dornase alfa for extracellular airway DNA hydrolysis

in the era of CFTR modulators. Expert Review of Respiratory Medicine. 2024:1-16. DOI: 10.1080/17476348.2024.2394694

[71] Montgomery ST, Mall MA, Kicic A, Stick SM. Hypoxia and sterile inflammation in cystic fibrosis airways: Mechanisms and potential therapies. European Respiratory Journal. 2017;**49**:1600903. DOI: 10.1183/13993003.00903-2016

[72] Page LK, Staples KJ, Spalluto CM, Watson A, Wilkinson TMA. Influence of hypoxia on the epithelial-pathogen interactions in the lung: Implications for respiratory disease. Frontiers in Immunology. 2021;**13**:653969. DOI: 10.3389/fimmu.2021.653969

[73] Shahriary CM, Chin TW, Nussbaum E. Respiratory epithelial cell lines exposed to anoxia produced inflammatory mediators. Anatomy & Cell Biology. 2012;**45**:221-228. DOI: 10.5115/acb.2012.45.4.221

[74] Chen Y, Gaber T. Hypoxia/HIF modulates immune responses. Biomediines. 2021;**9**:260. DOI: 10.3390/biomedicines9030260

Chapter 3

Utilization of Medicinal Herbal Plants in the Management of Respiratory Conditions

Ruchika Garg, Kiran Dobhal and Alka Singh

Abstract

This chapter examines the therapeutic powers of herbal medicinal plants in treating long-term respiratory diseases like bronchitis, asthma, and chronic obstructive pulmonary disease (COPD). Millions worldwide suffer from chronic respiratory disorders, which are a major cause of morbidity and mortality. Medicinal interventions are often used in conventional therapies to reduce symptoms and manage the condition. However, herbal medicinal plants offer an alternative method by utilizing their bioactive ingredients and traditional knowledge. The chapter reviews the literature and research on the effectiveness and mechanisms of the action of several herbal medicinal plants in treating respiratory diseases, including their effects on the immune system, mucolytic activity, bronchodilation, antioxidants, and inflammation. Several herbal plants show promise in treatment, such as ginseng, astragalus, marshmallow root, mullein, turmeric, ginger, liqorice, eucalyptus, peppermint, thyme, green tea, oregano, rosemary, and marshmallow root. They aid in symptom alleviation, immune response modulation, mucus clearance, oxidative stress reduction, inflammation reduction, and airway enlargement. In conclusion, herbal medicinal plants are essential for comprehensive care of long-term respiratory conditions, providing a multitude of therapeutic choices with varying mechanisms of action and potential advantages.

Keywords: herbal medicines, respiratory diseases, turmeric, eucalyptus, liqorice, anti-inflammatory, bronchodilation

1. Introduction

The ancient knowledge of herbal medicine has woven itself through the fabric of human existence for millennia, offering remarkable insights into managing and treating various ailments. Among these ailments, respiratory conditions have long warranted the attention of healers and herbalists alike [1]. From bronchitis to asthma, the breath is both a vital sign of life and a delicate thread susceptible to environmental, physiological, and emotional strains [2]. Fortunately, many medicinal plants have emerged as allies in nurturing lung health, revealing a profound synergy between nature's bounty and human well-being. Certain plants have gained recognition for their therapeutic properties in the shadows of towering trees and among the gentle rustle of herbs. The first among these, perhaps, is the humble thyme (*Thymus vulgaris*). Revered for its antiseptic and anti-inflammatory qualities, thyme has been utilized for centuries to relieve coughs and bronchial congestion [2]. Its active compounds, thymol, and carvacrol, work to relax the muscles of the respiratory tract, promoting easier breathing and providing relief from the discomfort of persistent coughs [3, 4].

This study explores the therapeutic properties of various plant species, particularly those used in treating respiratory diseases. Over 35,000 plant species are used globally, especially in emerging countries where traditional medicine, primarily plant-based pharmaceuticals, is a primary healthcare resource [5]. Medicinal plants like aloe, ginger, turmeric, tulsi, and neem are used to treat various respiratory ailments. These plants contain bioactive compounds like tannins, alkaloids, sugars, terpenoids, steroids, and flavonoids, which have diverse therapeutic applications. Some plants, like *Echinacea purpurea* and *Zingiber officinale*, have potential for adjuvant symptomatic therapy in respiratory conditions like COPD, bronchitis, asthma, and the common cold. This review provides valuable insights for researchers in herbal medicine, suggesting these plants could be novel therapeutic agents for respiratory diseases [6]. Equally, the potent elderflower (*Sambucus nigra*) has established its place in the repertoire of herbal remedies. A diaphoretic and expectorant elderflower engages with the body's natural processes; its flowers, when brewed into a tea or utilized in tinctures, help open the airways and dissolve mucus, easing symptoms of colds and flu. The slightly sweet and floral undertones of elderflower tea offer not just relief but also a moment of tranquility amidst the chaos of respiratory distress [7–10].

Linden (Tilia spp.), cherished for its calming properties, has also been a staple in the management of respiratory complaints [11]. Laced with calming flavonoids, linden's flowers are often steeped to create balmy infusions, which can soothe the throat while aiding in the expulsion of phlegm. As one savors the warmth of the herbal infusion, linden grants a necessary reprieve during the trials of respiratory illness, bridging the gap between physical relief and emotional comfort. As the seasons turn, so too do the array of plants practitioners turn to. Licorice root (*Glycyrrhiza glabra*), with its sweet flavor and deeply held medicinal virtues, has a particular affinity for the respiratory system. Acting as a demulcent, licorice creates a protective layer along mucous membranes, mitigating irritation and inflammation. Its synergistic qualities hinge on a delicate balance, elucidating the importance of understanding the individual needs of each patient [12, 13].

Peppermint (Mentha × Piperita), with its refreshing scent and cooling properties, has also proven beneficial. The menthol within peppermint oil serves not only to open the airways but also imparts a pleasant relief, allowing one to breathe more deeply when the discomfort of congestion looms large. In many home remedies, peppermint is a favorite for inhalation or steam treatments, where its volatile oils lift spirits and clear the path for unobstructed breathing [14]. Equipped with the wisdom of these herbal remedies, it is crucial to consider their applications in a comprehensive approach to respiratory health. The infusion of traditional plant-based therapies amidst modern techniques forms a holistic strategy, cultivating a space where patients feel empowered and informed. Each individual responds differently to herbal treatments; therefore, personalized care, guided by knowledgeable practitioners, remains a cornerstone of effective management [15].

Despite the promise shown by herbal medicine, it is essential to reconcile its use within the framework of evidence-based practices. Continued research is needed to unveil these plants' intricacies and interactions with the human body. As scientific inquiry advances, there remains an enduring belief that the wisdom of the ancients holds a place in contemporary health discussions. In the ever-evolving narrative of health and illness, the exploitation of medicinal herbal plants offers a pathway rich with potential. Each breath we take resonates with the knowledge that nature surrounds us that healing is not merely a product of science but an embrace of the wisdom that has guided humanity through ages gone by. To turn toward herbal remedies in managing respiratory conditions is to open oneself to the serene embrace of nature's enduring legacy, reminding us of the intricate connections between our lives and the world of botanical healing beyond. Commonly used to treat pneumonia, bronchitis, asthma, colds, and coughs are the leaves of medicinal plants such as Acacia torta, *Ocimum sanctum* (OS), Menthahaplocalyx, Lactucavirosa, Convolvulus pluricaulis, and Acalyphaindica [16].

2. Herbal preparation

The plants mentioned are indeed used in various traditional medicine systems for treating respiratory conditions. Here is a brief overview of each, including their common uses and forms in **Figure 1**.

2.1 Acacia torta

Common name: Torta Acacia.

Uses: Traditionally used in some cultures for its potential anti-inflammatory and expectorant properties. It is less commonly cited in modern herbal medicine, but it might be used for respiratory support based on local practices.

Forms: Typically used in decoctions or infusions [17].

2.2 *Ocimum sanctum*

Common name: Holy Basil or Tulsi.

Uses: Known for its adaptogenic, anti-inflammatory, and antimicrobial properties. Holy Basil is commonly used in Ayurvedic medicine to support respiratory health, relieve coughs, and help with asthma shown in (**Figure 1**).

Forms: Tea, tincture, capsules, or fresh leaves [17–20].

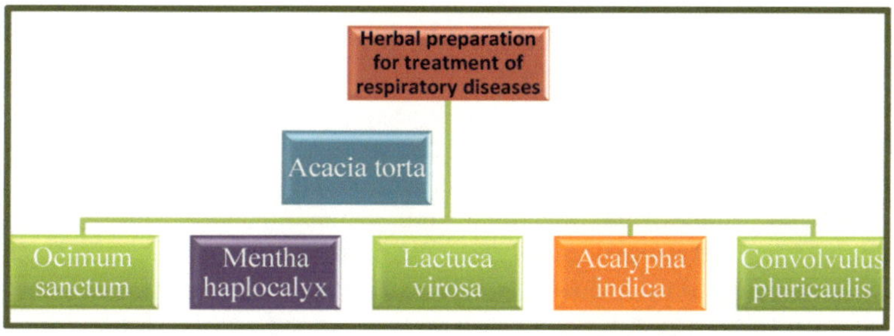

Figure 1.
Herbal preparation for treatment of Respiratory diseases.

2.3 Mentha haplocalyx

Common name: Spearmint.

Uses: Spearmint is used for its soothing effects on the respiratory tract and its potential to relieve coughs and colds. It has mild antispasmodic and expectorant properties.

Forms: Tea, essential oil, or fresh leaves [21].

2.4 *Lactuca virosa*

Common name: Wild Lettuce.

Uses: Often used traditionally as a sedative and cough suppressant. It has been used in folk medicine to treat coughs, bronchitis, and other respiratory issues.

Forms: Tea, tincture, or capsules [22].

2.5 Convolvulus pluricaulis

Common name: Shankhapushpi.

Uses: Known for its use in Ayurvedic medicine as a brain tonic, it is also used for respiratory conditions due to its potential anti-inflammatory and expectorant effects.

Forms: Tea, powder, or capsules [23].

2.6 *Acalypha indica*

Common name: Indian Acalypha.

Uses: Used in traditional medicine systems for its potential anti-inflammatory, expectorant, and antimicrobial properties. It is used for respiratory issues such as coughs and bronchitis.

Forms: Decoctions, infusions, or topical applications [24].

These plants have been traditionally used in various cultures, but modern scientific research on their effectiveness and safety might be limited. Combining herbal remedies with conventional treatments and professional guidance can offer a balanced approach to managing respiratory conditions.

3. Herbal preparations for treating respiratory conditions

3.1 Herbal preparations have been used for centuries to support respiratory health: Here are some commonly used herbs and preparation for curing the respiratory infection

3.1.1 Eucalyptus (Eucalyptus globulus)

Forms: Essential oil, tea, lozenges [23–25].

Uses: Eucalyptus, particularly *Eucalyptus globulus* (blue gum), has been traditionally used for its medicinal properties, especially in treating respiratory conditions. The active compounds in eucalyptus, such as *eucalyptol (cineole),* have demonstrated various therapeutic effects that can benefit those suffering from respiratory issues. Known for its decongestant and anti-inflammatory properties, eucalyptus can help relieve symptoms of colds, coughs, and bronchitis as shown in **Table 1** [34].

Herb	Primary benefits	Mechanism of action	Common uses
Echinacea (*Echinacea purpurea*)	Immune system support	Stimulates white blood cell activity	Cold prevention, respiratory infections
Elderberry (*Sambucus nigra*)	Immune system support, antiviral	Contains antioxidants and vitamins	Flu and cold symptom relief
Thyme (*Thymus vulgaris*)	Mucolytic, antimicrobial	Contains thymol and carvacrol	Cough, bronchitis, and mucus clearance
Marshmallow root (*Althaea officinalis*)	Mucolytic, soothing	Contains mucilage	Soothing throat, cough relief
Ginger (*Zingiber officinale*)	Bronchodilator, anti-inflammatory	Contains gingerol	Asthma management, cough relief
Ephedra (*Ephedra sinica*)	Bronchodilator	Contains ephedrine	Asthma, bronchial congestion
Green Tea (*Camellia sinensis*)	Antioxidant	Contains catechins (EGCG)	Respiratory health support, overall antioxidant
Turmeric (*Curcuma longa*)	Anti-inflammatory, antioxidant	Contains curcumin	Inflammation reduction, respiratory health
Holy Basil (*Ocimum sanctum*)	Anti-inflammatory, adaptogenic	Reduces inflammation and stress	Asthma, chronic respiratory issues
Boswellia (*Boswellia serrata*)	Anti-inflammatory	Contains boswellic acids	Chronic inflammation, asthma

Table 1.
Summary of herbs commonly used in respiratory diseases, categorized by their primary benefits and effects: [26–33].

How to use eucalyptus for respiratory relief:

a. *Steam inhalation*: Add a few drops of eucalyptus oil to a bowl of hot water and inhale the steam for 10–15 minutes.

b. *Diffuser*: Use a diffuser with eucalyptus oil to purify the air and ease breathing difficulties.

c. *Chest rubs*: Apply diluted eucalyptus oil (mixed with carrier oil, like coconut or olive oil) to the chest and neck area to ease congestion and soothe coughing.

d. *Hot compress*: Soak a cloth in hot water with eucalyptus oil and apply it to the chest or back to relieve congestion.

3.1.2 Thyme (*Thymus vulgaris*)

Forms: Tea, tincture, essential oil.

Uses: Thyme (*Thymus vulgaris*) has a long history of use in traditional medicine, particularly for its beneficial effects on the respiratory system. Its medicinal properties are largely attributed to compounds such as thymol, carvacrol, and other essential oils, which have antimicrobial, expectorant, and anti-inflammatory effects. Thyme has antibacterial and expectorant properties, which can help with coughs and respiratory infections and utilized in traditional medicine for treating respiratory diseases like asthma and bronchitis, as well as other pathologies due to their antiseptic, antispasmodic, antitussive, antimicrobial, antifungal, antioxidant, and antiviral properties [26].

How to use thyme for respiratory health:

a. *Thyme tea*: Steep 1–2 teaspoons of dried thyme leaves in boiling water for about 10 minutes. Drink this tea up to 2–3 times per day to help with coughing, bronchitis, or other respiratory issues.

b. *Thyme steam inhalation*: Add a few drops of thyme essential oil or a handful of dried thyme to hot water and inhale the steam to relieve chest congestion or sinus issues.

c. *Thyme syrup*: You can make a thyme syrup by boiling thyme in water with honey. This can be a soothing remedy for coughs and sore throats.

3.1.3 Peppermint (Mentha piperita)

Forms: Tea, essential oil, lozenges.

Uses: Another herb that is frequently used for respiratory health is peppermint (*Mentha piperita*), which has calming and healing qualities. Some of its main active ingredients, including menthol, have many respiratory system advantages. The benefits of peppermint include clearing congestion, opening up the airways, and easing the symptoms of coughs, colds, and respiratory ailments including bronchitis and asthma. Peppermint contains menthol, which can help soothe the throat and ease coughing, as well as act as a decongestant [27].

3.1.4 Licorice root (Glycyrrhiza glabra)

Forms: Tea, tincture, capsules.

Uses: *Glycyrrhiza glabra*, or liquorice root, has been used for millennia in traditional medicine by many different civilisations, especially in Asia and Europe, because of its many medicinal benefits, which include supporting respiratory health. The therapeutic properties of the root are attributed to a number of active substances, including glycyrrhizin, flavonoids, and saponins. Licorice root is known for its demulcent and expectorant properties, which can help soothe irritated mucous membranes and promote the expulsion of mucus [27].

3.1.5 Ginger (Zingiber officinale)

Forms: Tea, capsules, fresh ginger.

Uses: *Zingiber officinale*, or ginger, is a potent root with many therapeutic uses that makes it a great option for promoting respiratory health. The active ingredients in ginger, including zingiberene, shogaol, and gingerol, are responsible for the plant's expectorant, antibacterial, anti-inflammatory, and immune-boosting effects. Ginger has anti-inflammatory and antioxidant properties, which can help alleviate symptoms of respiratory infections and improve overall lung function [27].

3.1.6 Marshmallow root (Althaea officinalis)

Forms: Tea, tincture, capsules.

Uses: The traditional herbal treatment marshmallow root (*Althaea officinalis*) is well-known for its calming effects, particularly on the respiratory system. Much of the root's medicinal impact comes from mucilage, a gelatinous material that gives the root its distinctively slippery feel. Since marshmallow root coats and protects mucous membranes, lowers inflammation, and speeds up healing, it has been used for generations to treat a variety of respiratory conditions. Marshmallow root is a mucilaginous herb that helps soothe and coat the respiratory tract, making it useful for dry coughs and sore throats [28].

3.1.7 Mullein (Verbascum thapsus)

Forms: Tea, tincture, capsules.

Uses: Mullein (*Verbascum thapsus*) is a powerful herb with a long history of use for respiratory health. Due to its calming, expectorant, and anti-inflammatory qualities, the plant has long been used to treat a range of lung and airway problems. Compounds found in its leaves, blossoms, and roots promote lung function, ease congestion, and open up airways. Mullein is used to soothe respiratory conditions, such as coughs and bronchitis, due to its expectorant and anti-inflammatory properties [28].

3.1.8 Lobelia (Lobelia inflata)

Forms: Tea, tincture, capsules.

Uses: Strong herb lobelia (*Lobelia inflata*) has long been used to promote respiratory health. Lobelia is well-known for its capacity to uplift and strengthen the respiratory system. Because of its bronchodilator and expectorant properties, it is very useful in the treatment of respiratory ailments like as bronchitis, asthma, and even nicotine withdrawal. Lobelia is a powerful herb that can act as a bronchial stimulant and expectorant, helping to clear mucus and ease breathing [28].

3.1.9 Slippery elm (Ulmus rubra)

Forms: Tea, powder, capsules.

Uses: The well-known plant slippery elm (*Ulmus rubra*) is highly valued for its calming and restorative qualities, especially for the respiratory system. Mucilage, found in the inner bark of slippery elm, is a potent demulcent that, when combined with water, takes the shape of a gel. This mucilage is very helpful for respiratory health since it may coat and soothe inflamed mucous membranes. Slippery elm contains mucilage, which can soothe the mucous membranes of the respiratory tract and alleviate coughs and sore throats.

3.1.10 Astragalus (Astragalus membranaceus)

Forms: Tea, tincture, capsules.

Uses: *Astragalus* (*Astragalus membranaceus*) is a powerful herb, often used in Traditional Chinese Medicine (TCM), and is highly regarded for its ability to enhance the immune system and support respiratory health. Astragalus has many benefits, particularly in bolstering the body's natural defenses, which makes it an excellent choice for preventing and managing respiratory conditions. While it is primarily used as an immune booster, its supportive actions on the respiratory system are noteworthy. Astragalus is known for its immune-boosting properties, which can help strengthen the body's defenses against respiratory infections [24–29].

3.2 Formulation of herbs

Teas: Steep the herb in hot water for about 10–15 minutes. This is a gentle way to ingest the herb and benefit from its properties.

Tinctures: Herbal tinctures are concentrated extracts. Follow the dosage instructions on the label.

Essential oils: Use essential oils cautiously. They can be inhaled via diffusers or applied topically when diluted with carrier oil [26, 29].

Capsules/tablets: Follow dosage instructions provided by the manufacturer or a healthcare provider.

3.3 Important considerations

a. *Consult with a healthcare provider*: Before starting any herbal remedy, especially if you are pregnant, nursing, or taking medications, it's important to consult with a healthcare provider.

b. *Allergies and interactions*: Be aware of potential allergic reactions and interactions with other medications or conditions.

c. *Quality*: Use high-quality, reputable sources for herbs to ensure safety and effectiveness. Ensure that you use herbs from reputable sources to avoid contaminants and ensure the efficacy of the treatment.

4. Herbal medicines have been used for centuries to treat respiratory conditions, and many of them are valued for their potential therapeutic benefits: Here is a comprehensive look at the benefits of herbal medicines for respiratory health, supported by research and traditional knowledge

4.1 Anti-inflammatory effects

Benefit: Many herbs have anti-inflammatory properties that can help reduce inflammation in the airways, making them useful for conditions like asthma and chronic bronchitis.

Examples:

Holy basil (Ocimum sanctum): Known for its anti-inflammatory and adaptogenic effects. Research has shown it can help reduce inflammation and oxidative stress in respiratory conditions [31].

Turmeric (Curcuma longa): Contains curcumin, which has been shown to have potent anti-inflammatory effects [32].

4.2 Antimicrobial and antiviral effects

Benefit: Some herbs possess antimicrobial or antiviral properties, which can help combat respiratory infections.

Examples:

Eucalyptus (Eucalyptus globulus): Has antimicrobial and antiviral properties, which can aid in treating respiratory infections and easing symptoms [34].

Thyme (Thymus vulgaris): Contains thymol, which has antimicrobial properties beneficial for respiratory infections [33].

4.3 Expectorant properties

Benefit: Herbal expectorants help loosen mucus and facilitate its expulsion from the respiratory tract, which is beneficial for conditions like bronchitis and chronic coughs.

Examples:

Mullein (Verbascum thapsus): Acts as an expectorant, helping to clear mucus from the lungs [35].

Licorice root (Glycyrrhiza glabra): Soothes the mucous membranes and helps in expelling mucus [36].

4.4 Bronchodilator effects

Benefit: Some herbs have bronchodilator properties, which can help open up the airways and improve breathing in conditions like asthma.

Examples:

Ephedra (Ephedra sinica): Traditionally used in Chinese medicine to relieve asthma and other respiratory conditions due to its bronchodilator effect [37, 38].

Ginger (Zingiber officinale): Has been shown to have bronchodilator effects and may help in managing asthma [39–41].

4.5 Antioxidant effects

Benefit: Antioxidant-rich herbs can help reduce oxidative stress in the respiratory tract, which can be beneficial in managing chronic respiratory diseases [42–44].

Examples:

Green tea (Camellia sinensis): Rich in antioxidants like catechins that can help reduce oxidative stress and inflammation [45].

Ginseng (Panax ginseng): Contains ginsenosides with antioxidant properties that may support respiratory health [37, 44].

4.6 Adaptogenic effects

Benefit: Adaptogens help the body adapt to stress and support overall health, which can be beneficial for individuals with chronic respiratory conditions exacerbated by stress.

Examples:

Holy basil (Ocimum sanctum): As an adaptogen, it helps reduce stress and inflammation, potentially benefiting respiratory health [45].

4.7 Soothing and demulcent effects

Benefit: Some herbs have soothing properties that can help alleviate throat irritation and cough [46].

Examples:

Marshmallow root (Althaea officinalis): Acts as a demulcent, soothing irritated mucous membrane [46–48].

Slippery elm (Ulmus rubra): Contains mucilage that coats and soothes the throat and respiratory tract.

4.8 Immune system support

Herbs that support the immune system can help enhance the body's defense mechanisms against infections and illnesses.

Benefit: Known for its immune-boosting properties. It can stimulate the activity of white blood cells and enhance overall immune response. Clinical studies have demonstrated its efficacy in treating influenza and respiratory infections.

Examples:

Echinacea (Echinacea purpurea): Studies have shown Echinacea can reduce the duration and severity of colds [49].

Elderberry (Sambucus nigra): Rich in antioxidants and vitamins, Elderberry is effective in reducing the severity and duration of flu symptoms [39, 49].

4.9 Mucolytic activity (mucus clearance)

Benefit: Herbs with mucolytic properties help to break down and expel mucus from the respiratory tract. Thyme has been shown to be effective in treating bronchitis and coughs due to its mucolytic properties. Contains mucilage, which forms a soothing layer on mucous membranes and helps in the clearance of mucus.

Thyme (Thymus vulgaris) Contains thymol and carvacrol, which have mucolytic and expectorant effects. It helps in loosening mucus and improving cough efficiency [50].

Marshmallow root (Althaea officinalis): The demulcent properties of marshmallow root make it effective in soothing irritated tissues and aiding in mucus expulsion [48].

4.10 Bronchodilation (airway opening)

Herbs that have bronchodilator effects can help open airways and improve breathing.

Ginger (Zingiber officinale).

Benefit: Contains gingerol and other compounds that have bronchodilatory effects, which can help in managing asthma and bronchitis [42].

Research: Ginger has been found to relax airway smooth muscle and improve airflow [36, 42].

Ephedra (Ephedra sinica).

Benefit: Known for its bronchodilator effects due to its active compound, ephedrine. It has been used traditionally to treat asthma and respiratory issues.

Research: Ephedra has shown effectiveness in opening airways and relieving symptoms of asthma [51].

5. Using herbal medicines (HM) for respiratory conditions can be beneficial, but it is important to exercise caution to ensure safety and effectiveness: Here are some key precautions to consider, along with references for further reading

5.1 Consultation with healthcare providers

Importance: Always consult with a healthcare provider before starting any herbal regimen, especially if you have pre-existing health conditions or are on other medications [51, 52]. Herbal medicines can interact with conventional drugs and may not be suitable for everyone [51].

5.2 Potential drug interactions

Risk: Herbal medicines can interact with prescription and over-the-counter medications, potentially altering their effectiveness or causing adverse effects (AE).

Example: Licorice root, used for its anti-inflammatory properties, can interact with antihypertensive drugs and increase blood pressure (BP) [51].

5.3 Quality and purity of herbal products

Importance: Ensure that the herbal products you use are sourced from reputable suppliers to avoid contamination with harmful substances or incorrect dosages [52].

5.4 Allergic reactions

Risk: Some individuals may experience allergic reactions to specific herbs. It is essential to start with a small dose and monitor for any adverse effects.

Example: Peppermint oil can cause allergic reactions or skin irritation in some people [53].

5.5 Dosage and duration

Importance: Follow recommended dosages and durations for herbal treatments to avoid potential toxicity or side effects. Overuse of certain herbs can lead to adverse effects.

Example: Excessive use of licorice root can lead to hypertension and hypokalemia [54, 55].

5.6 Pregnancy and lactation

Caution: Pregnant and lactating women should use herbal medicines with caution, as some herbs may affect fetal development or be excreted in breast milk.

Example: Eucalyptus oil is generally considered safe in small amounts but should be used cautiously [56, 57].

5.7 Underlying health conditions

Risk: Individuals with chronic health conditions such as diabetes, hypertension, or liver disease should be particularly cautious, as herbal remedies might exacerbate these conditions.

Example: Herbal supplements like licorice can affect blood sugar levels and interact with diabetes medications [58].

5.8 Scientific evidence and efficacy

Importance: Use herbal remedies supported by scientific evidence to ensure they are effective for the intended use [53].

5.9 Efficacy and safety

Depending on how they are prepared and how much is taken, herbal treatments may or may not be effective. To ensure efficacy and safety, standardization and quality control are essential.

5.10 Side effects and interactions

There may be interactions and side effects between herbal treatments and medications. Before beginning any herbal treatment, it is important to see a healthcare provider, particularly for individuals with long-term respiratory disorders or other health concerns [56].

Although many herbal medications have encouraging evidence for treating respiratory diseases, further study is necessary to definitively confirm their safety and efficacy, especially large-scale clinical studies. Before taking a natural remedy, always get medical advice [58–61].

6. Conclusion

Herbal medicines offer various benefits for respiratory health, including anti-inflammatory, expectorant, antimicrobial, bronchodilator, antioxidant, soothing, and adaptogenic effects. While many herbs have demonstrated efficacy in managing respiratory conditions, it is important to use them responsibly and in conjunction with conventional medical treatments. Always consult with healthcare providers before starting any new herbal regimen (HR), especially if you have existing health conditions or are taking other medications. Herbal remedies can be a valuable complement to conventional treatments, but they should be used thoughtfully and in conjunction with professional medical advice. HM can be effective for managing respiratory conditions, but they should be used with caution like Astragalus (*Astragalus membranaceus*) is an excellent herb for supporting respiratory health due to its immune-enhancing, anti-inflammatory, and lung-supportive properties, and Slippery elm is an excellent herb for respiratory health, especially for soothing sore throats, reducing coughing, and promoting the healing of irritated airways. Always consult with healthcare professionals, be aware of potential interactions, and use high-quality products to ensure safety and efficacy. Herbal medicines have been used for centuries to treat respiratory conditions, and many of them are valued for their potential therapeutic benefits. Here is a comprehensive look at the benefits of herbal medicines for respiratory health, supported by research and traditional knowledge. Since ancient times, herbal remedies have been utilized to treat respiratory disorders, and a growing amount of scientific research is demonstrating their effectiveness.

Acknowledgements

Authors conveyed special thanks to Mr. Suresh Gupta, Chairman of Maharaja Agrasen University, Baddi, Solan, H.P., for encouraging publishing this review work. Authors also acknowledge the use of Quillbot software tool was used for language polishing of the manuscript.

Author contribution

RG drafted as well as wrote the manuscript. KD significantly revised all the manuscript and improved the data that were involved in the study design. AS reviewed all data collection, data management, and accept responsibility for the overall content as a guarantor. RG approved the version to be published. All authors approved the final manuscript.

Funding

None.

Conflict of interest

The authors declare no conflict of interest.

Patient and public involvement

None declared.

Abbreviation

AE	adverse effect
BP	blood pressure
COPD	chronic obstructive pulmonary diseases
EGCG	epigallocatechin gallate
HM	herbal medicines
HR	herbal regimen
OS	*Occimum sanctum*

Author details

Ruchika Garg[1*], Kiran Dobhal[2] and Alka Singh[3]

1 School of Pharmacy, Maharaja Agrasen University, Baddi, India

2 Shivalik College of Pharmacy, Dehradun, Uttarakhand, India

3 School of Pharmacy, Sardar Bhagwan Singh University, Dehradun, India

*Address all correspondence to: aggrwal.nov24@gmail.com

References

[1] Wachtel-Galor S, Benzie IFF. Herbal medicine: An introduction to its history, usage, regulation, current trends, and research needs. In: Benzie IFF, Wachtel-Galor S, editors. Herbal Medicine: Biomolecular and Clinical Aspects. 2nd ed. Boca Raton (FL): CRC Press/Taylor & Francis; 2011. Ch1. Available from: https://www.ncbi.nlm.nih.gov/books/NBK92773/

[2] Garg R, Piplani M, Upadhayay A, Singh Y, Bhateja P. A review on comparison of allopathic medicines to other drug therapies in the management of asthma. Infectious Disorders-Drug Targets (Formerly Current Drug Targets-Infectious Disorders). 2024;**24**(2):1-12. DOI: 10.2174/0118715265249796231018050521

[3] Garg R, Piplani M, Singh Y, Bhateja P, Rana R. An overview of integrated risk factors with prevention and prevalence of asthma at the global level. Current Traditional Medicine. 2024;**10**(4):71-81. DOI: 10.2174/2215083810666230525153908

[4] Garg R, Piplani M, Singh Y, Joshi Y. Epidemiology, pathophysiology, and pharmacological status of asthma. Current Respiratory Medicine Reviews. 2022;**18**(4):247-258. DOI: 10.2174/1573398X18666220526164329

[5] Firdaus A, Yunus MH, Izhar SK, Afaq U. Medicinal plants in the treatment of respiratory diseases and their future aspects. Recent Patents on Biotechnology. 2025;**19**(1):2-18. DOI: 10.2174/0118722083278561231212072408

[6] Kim HP, Lim H, Kwon YS. Therapeutic potential of medicinal plants and their constituents on lung inflammatory disorders. Biomolecules & Therapeutics. 2017;**25**(2):91. DOI: 10.4062/biomolther.2016.187

[7] Webmd [Internet]. Elderflower Uses, Side effects, and more. 2024. Available from: https://www.webmd.com/vitamins/ai/ingredientmono-708/elderflower [Accessed: September 15, 2024]

[8] Tabaszewska M, Sikora E. The effect of the plant stabilisation method on the composition and antioxidant properties of elderflower (*Sambucus nigra* L.). extract. Molecules. 2023;**28**(5):2365. DOI: 10.3390/molecules28052365

[9] Uhl KR, Mitchell AE. Headspace volatile organic and phenolic compounds in elderflowers and elderflower teas of blue elderberry (*Sambucus nigra* ssp. cerulea). ACS Food Science & Technology. 2022;**2**(10):1535-1545. DOI: 10.1021/acsfoodscitech.2c00177

[10] Tabaszewska M, Sikora E. The effect of the plant stabilisation method on the composition and antioxidant properties of elderflower (Sambucus nigra L.) extract. Molecules. 2023;**28**(5):2365, 1-11. DOI: 10.3390/molecules28052365

[11] Toker G, Küpeli E, Memisoğlu M, Yesilada E. Flavonoids with antinociceptive and anti-inflammatory activities from the leaves of Tilia argentea (silver linden). Journal of Ethnopharmacology. 2004;**95**(2-3):393-397. DOI: 10.1016/j.jep

[12] Yeh CF, Wang KC, Chiang LC, Shieh DE, Yen MH, San CJ. Water extract of licorice had anti-viral activity against human respiratory syncytial virus in human respiratory tract cell lines. Journal of Ethnopharmacology.

2013;**148**(2):466-473. DOI: 10.1016/j.jep.2013.04.040

[13] Taniguchi H, Terayama T, Kiriu N, Kato H, Seno S, Sekine Y, et al. Case report: Severe respiratory failure caused by licorice. Frontiers in Pharmacology. 2023;**14**:1289755. DOI: 10.3389/fphar

[14] Hudz N, Kobylinska L, Pokajewicz K, Horčinová Sedláčková V, Fedin R, Voloshyn M, et al. Mentha piperita: Essential oil and extracts, their biological activities, and perspectives on the development of new medicinal and cosmetic products. Molecules. 2023;**28**(21):7444. DOI: 10.3390/molecules28217444

[15] Wang H, Chen Y, Wang L, Liu Q, Yang S, Wang C. Advancing herbal medicine: Enhancing product quality and safety through robust quality control practices. Frontiers in Pharmacology. 2023;**14**:1265178. DOI: 10.3389/fphar

[16] Taur DJ, Patil RY. Some medicinal plants with antiasthmatic potential: A current status. Asian Pacific Journal of Tropical Biomedicine. 2011;**1**(5):413-418. DOI: 10.1016/S2221-1691(11)60091-9

[17] Cohen MM. Tulsi-*Ocimum sanctum*: A herb for all reasons. Journal of Ayurveda and Integrative Medicine. 2014;**4**:251. DOI: 10.4103/0975-9476.146554

[18] Joshi Y, Garg R, Juyal D. Evaluation of synergistic antimicrobial activity of Gemifloxacin with *Linum usitatissimum* seed oil. Liver. 2014;**2**(4):384-388. DOI: 10.31254/phyto.2014.3602

[19] Saha S, Prinsa VJ, Mahato AK, Srivastava S, Dobhal K, Kawsar SM. In silico assessment of the role of iridoid in the treatment of Zika and influenza virus infection. The Philippine Journal of Science. 2023;**152**(5):1953-1958. DOI: 10.56899/152.05.35

[20] Villena-Tejada M, Vera-Ferchau I, Cardona-Rivero A, Zamalloa-Cornejo R, Quispe-Florez M, Frisancho-Triveño Z, et al. Use of medicinal plants for COVID-19 prevention and respiratory symptom treatment during the pandemic in Cusco, Peru: A cross-sectional survey. PLoS One. 2021;**16**(9):e0257165, 4918-4929

[21] He XF, Geng CA, Huang XY, Ma YB, Zhang XM, Chen JJ. Chemical constituents from *Mentha haplocalyx* Briq. (*Mentha canadensis* L.) and their α-glucosidase inhibitory activities. Natural Products and Bioprospecting. 2019;**9**:223-229. DOI: 10.1007/s13659-019-0207-0

[22] Shi M, Gu J, Wu H, Rauf A, Emran TB, Khan Z, et al. Phytochemicals, nutrition, metabolism, bioavailability, and health benefits in lettuce-A comprehensive review. Antioxidants (Basel). 2022;**11**(6):1158, 1-23. DOI: 10.3390/antiox11061158

[23] Agarwa P, Sharma B, Fatima A, Jain SK. An update on ayurvedic herb convolvulus pluricaulis choisy. Asian Pacific Journal of Tropical Biomedicine. 2014;**4**(3):245-252. DOI: 10.1016/S2221-1691(14)60240-9

[24] Ninave PB, Patil SD. Pharmacological screening of *Acalypha indica* L.: Possible role in the treatment of asthma. Journal of Ethnopharmacology. 2022;**290**:115093. DOI: 10.1016/j.jep.2022.115093

[25] Pranskuniene Z, Balciunaite R, Simaitiene Z, Bernatoniene J. Herbal medicine uses for respiratory system disorders and possible trends in new herbal medicinal recipes during COVID-19 in Pasvalys district, Lithuania. International Journal of Environmental Research

and Public Health. 2022;**19**(15):8905. DOI: 10.3390/ijerph19158905

[26] Dauqan E, Abdullah A. Medicinal and functional values of thyme (*Thymus vulgaris* L.) herb. Journal Of Applied Biology & Biotechnology. 2017;**2**:17-22. DOI: 10.7324/JABB.2017.50203

[27] Armutcu F, Kucukbayrak A. Herbal remedies for respiratory tract infections. Infectious Diseases. 2021;**5**:46-71. DOI: 10.2174/9781681089225121050004

[28] Sultana S, Khan A, Safhi MM, Alhazmi HA. Cough suppressant herbal drugs: A review. International Journal of Pharmaceutical Science Invention. 2016;**5**:15-28

[29] Villena-Tejada M, Vera-Ferchau I, Cardona-Rivero A, Zamalloa-Cornejo R, Quispe-Florez M, Frisancho-Triveño Z, et al. Use of medicinal plants for COVID-19 prevention and respiratory symptom treatment during the pandemic in Cusco, Peru: A cross-sectional survey. PLoS One. 2021;**16**(9):e0257165, 1-18

[30] Shawarb N, Badrasawi M, Qaoud HA, Hussein F. An ethno-botanical study of medicinal plants used for the management of respiratory tract disorders in northern parts of Palestine. BMC Complementary Medicine and Therapies. 2023;**23**(1):387. DOI: 10.1186/s12906-023-04176-5

[31] Hudz N, Makowicz E, Shanaida M, Białoń M, Jasicka-Misiak I, Yezerska O, et al. Phytochemical evaluation of tinctures and essential oil obtained from *Satureja montana* herb. Molecules. 2020;**25**(20):4763. DOI: 10.3390/molecules25204763

[32] Prasad S, Aggarwal BB. Turmeric, the Golden Spice. Herbal Medicine: Biomolecular and Clinical Aspects. 2nd ed. Boca Raton (FL): CRC Press/Taylor; 2011. Available from: https://www.ncbi.nlm.nih.gov/books/NBK92752

[33] Borugă O, Jianu C, Mişcă C, Goleţ I, Gruia AT, Horhat FG. *Thymus vulgaris* essential oil: Chemical composition and antimicrobial activity. Journal of Medicine and Life. 2014;**7**(Spec Iss 3):56

[34] Jie S et al. Effects of different doses of eucalyptus oil from *Eucalyptus globulus* Labill on respiratory tract immunity and immune function in healthy rats. Frontiers in Pharmacology. 2020;**11**:1287. DOI: 10.3389/fphar.2020.01287

[35] Blanco-Salas J, Hortigón-Vinagre MP, Morales-Jadán D, Ruiz-Téllez T. Searching for scientific explanations for the uses of Spanish folk medicine: A review on the case of mullein (*Verbascum*, *Scrophulariaceae*). Biology (Basel). 2021;**10**(7):618. DOI: 10.3390/biology10070618

[36] Sigurjónsdóttir HÁ, Franzson L, Manhem K, Ragnarsson J, Sigurdsson G, Wallerstedt S. Liquorice-induced rise in blood pressure: A linear dose-response relationship. Journal of Human Hypertension. 2001;**15**(8):549-552. DOI: 10.1038/sj.jhh.1001215

[37] Jo EH, Jo IJ, Park SJ, Jo SH, Park MC. Effects of Ephedra sinica (ES) extract on the ovalbumin-induced allergid asthma in mice. The Journal of Korean Medicine Ophthalmology and Otolaryngology and Dermatology. 2014;**27**(3):84-95. DOI: 10.6114/jkood.2014.27.3.084 ·

[38] Manayi A, Vazirian M, Saeidnia S. *Echinacea purpurea*: Pharmacology, phytochemistry and analysis methods. Pharmacognosy Reviews. 2015;**9**(17):63. DOI: 10.4103/0973-7847.156353

[39] Zakay-Rones Z, Thom E, Wollan T, Wadstein J. Randomized study

of the efficacy and safety of oral elderberry extract in the treatment of influenza A and B virus infections. Journal of International Medical Research. 2004;**32**(2):132-140. DOI: 10.1177/147323000403200205

[40] Račková L, Cupáková M, Ťažký A, Mičová J, Kolek E, Košťálová D. Redox properties of ginger extracts: Perspectives of use of Zingiber officinale Rosc. as antidiabetic agent. Interdisciplinary Toxicology. 2013;**6**(1):26-33. DOI: 10.2478/intox-2013-0005

[41] Townsend EA, Siviski ME, Zhang Y, Xu C, Hoonjan B, Emala CW. Effects of ginger and its constituents on airway smooth muscle relaxation and calcium regulation. American Journal of Respiratory Cell and Molecular Biology. 2013;**48**(2):157-163. DOI: 10.1165/rcmb.2012-0231OC

[42] Rai M, Bhattarai S, Feitosa CM. Ch1. In: Ethnopharmacology of Wild Plants. 1st ed. Boca Raton: CRC Press; 2021. p. 426. DOI: 10.1201/9781003052814

[43] Cermelli C, Fabio A, Fabio G, Quaglio P. Effect of eucalyptus essential oil on respiratory bacteria and viruses. Current Microbiology. 2008;**56**(1):89-92. DOI: 10.1007/s00284-007-9045-0

[44] Paur I, Carlsen MH, Halvorsen BL, Blomhoff R. Antioxidants in herbs and spices: Roles in oxidative stress and redox signaling, Ch 2. In: Benzie IFF, Wachtel-Galor S, editors. Herbal Medicine: Biomolecular and Clinical Aspects. 2nd ed. Boca Raton (FL): CRC Press/Taylor & Francis; 2011

[45] Panossian A, Wikman G. Effects of adaptogens on the central nervous system and the molecular mechanisms associated with their stress-protective activity. Pharmaceuticals (Basel). 2010;**3**(1):188-224. DOI: 10.3390/ph3010188

[46] Mokra D, Adamcakova J, Mokry J. Greenteapolyphenol(−)-Epigallocatechin-3-Gallate (EGCG): A time for a new player in the treatment of respiratory diseases? Antioxidants (Basel). 2022;**11**(8):1566. DOI: 10.3390/antiox11081566

[47] Mahboubi M. Marsh mallow (*Althaea officinalis* L.) and its potency in the treatment of cough. Echter Eibisch (*Althaea officinalis* L.) und seine Wirksamkeit in der Behandlung von Husten. Complementary Medicine Research. 2020;**27**(3):174-183. DOI: 10.1159/000503747

[48] Bonaterra GA, Bronischewski K, Hunold P, et al. Anti-inflammatory and anti-oxidative effects of Phytohustil® and root extract of *Althaea officinalis* L. on macrophages in vitro. Frontiers in Pharmacology. 2020;**11**:290. DOI: 10.3389/fphar.2020.00290

[49] Block KI, Mead MN. Immune system effects of echinacea, ginseng, and astragalus: A review. Integrative Cancer Therapies. 2003;**2**(3):247-267. DOI: 10.1177/1534735403256419

[50] Kowalczyk A, Przychodna M, Sopata S, Bodalska A, Fecka I. Thymol and thyme essential oil-new insights into selected therapeutic applications. Molecules. 2020;**25**(18):4125. DOI: 10.3390/molecules25184125

[51] Tinkelman DG, Avner SE. Ephedrine therapy in asthmatic children. Clinical tolerance and absence of side effects. Journal of the American Medical Association. 1977;**237**(6):553-557

[52] Izzo AA. Interactions between herbs and conventional drugs: Overview of

the clinical data. Medical Principles and Practice. 2012;**21**(5):404-428. DOI: 10.1159/000334488

[53] Hammer KA, Carson CF, Riley TV. Antimicrobial activity of essential oils and other plant extracts. Journal of Applied Microbiology. 1999;**86**(6): 985-990. DOI: 10.1046/j.1365-2672.1999.00780.x

[54] Ekor M. The growing use of herbal medicines: Issues relating to adverse reactions and challenges in monitoring safety. Frontiers in Pharmacology. 2014;**4**:177. DOI: 10.3389/fphar.2013.00177

[55] Gurib-Fakim A. Medicinal plants: Traditions of yesterday and drugs of tomorrow. Molecular Aspects of Medicine. 2006;**27**(1):1-93. DOI: 10.1016/j.mam.2005.07.008

[56] Guo R, Pittler MH, Ernst E. Herbal medicines for the treatment of allergic rhinitis: A systematic review. Annals of Allergy, Asthma & Immunology. 2007;**99**(6):483. DOI: 95.:10.1016/S1081-1206(10)60375-4

[57] Kennedy DO, Scholey AB, Wesnes KA. Dose dependent changes in cognitive performance and mood following acute administration of ginseng to healthy young volunteers. Nutritional Neuroscience. 2001;**4**(4):295-310. DOI: 10.1080/1028415x.2001.11747370

[58] John LJ, Shantakumari N. Herbal medicines use during pregnancy: A review from the Middle East. Oman Medical Journal. 2015;**30**(4):229-236. DOI: 10.5001/omj.2015.48

[59] Cass H, Cott J. Herbal medicine. In: Handbook of Complementary and Alternative Therapies in Mental Health. Academic Press; 2002. pp. 377-400

[60] Tilburt JC, Kaptchuk TJ. Herbal medicine research and global health: An ethical analysis. Bulletin of the World Health Organization. 2008;**86**:594-599

[61] Kumar R, Singh Y, Piplani M, Bhateja P, Kumar G. Brijesh chemistry and pharmacological study of *Copaifera* spp. Ch. 4. In: Oils Is in Process in an International Book. Vol. 4. Bentham Science Publishers; 2024. pp. 79-108. DOI: 10.2174/9789815196832124040006

Chapter 4

Endoplasmic Reticulum Stress in Chronic Obstructive Pulmonary Disease

Tugba Raika Kıran

Abstract

Chronic obstructive pulmonary disease (COPD) is a long-term and worsening lung condition that results in irreversible damage to the airways and lung tissue, causing difficulty in breathing. The development of COPD is contributed to by cellular senescence, inflammation, protease-antiprotease imbalance, epigenetic changes, oxidative stress, endoplasmic reticulum (ER) stress, mitochondrial dysfunction, apoptosis, and cell death. Endoplasmic reticulum stress and cellular protein homeostasis are critical processes for maintaining the healthy function of cells. In response to ER stress, cells initiate a protective process called the unfolded protein response (UPR). Endoplasmic reticulum stress and UPR activation in the airways can be triggered by cigarette smoke, air pollution, bacteria, viruses, or other pathogenic microorganisms. In chronic diseases like COPD, persistent inflammation and oxidative stress can increase ER stress. This can cause continuous activation of UPR mechanisms, which can impair cell function. Chronic ER stress and insufficient protein homeostasis can lead to apoptosis and harm to lung tissue. The disruption of these vital processes, which are crucial for maintaining healthy cell functions, is a key factor in the development of chronic conditions such as COPD. Regulation of ER stress and maintaining protein balance may be a potential target for managing these diseases.

Keywords: chronic obstructive pulmonary disease, ER stress, unfolded protein response pathways, apoptosis, inflammation

1. Introduction

Chronic obstructive pulmonary disease (COPD), a worldwide health issue associated with significant morbidity and mortality, is a persistent inflammatory lung condition that leads to restricted airflow from the lungs [1]. One of the most widespread causes is long-term exposure to irritating gases or particulate pollutants from cigarette smoke [2]. Other causes include the use of biofuels in poorly ventilated areas, chemicals used in building construction, indoor pollutants such as radon gas emitted from the ground, and airborne biological pollutants, such as mold, dust mites, and mildew [3]. In a global study evaluating COPD participants who have never smoked, it has been reported that approximately 25–40% of all COPD cases are due to factors other than tobacco smoking [4]. Genetic polymorphisms in the genes coding for α1-antitrypsin (AAT), α1-antichymotrypsin (AACT), α2-macroglobulin (A2M), matrix metalloproteinases (MMP), serine protease inhibitor 1 (SeRPINA1), serine protease inhibitor 2 (SeRPINA2), microsomal epoxide hydrolase 1 (EPHX1), glutathione S-transferase (GST), heme oxygenase-1 (HMOX1), cytochrome P4501A1 (CYP1A1), vitamin D-binding protein (VDBP), tumor necrosis factor-α (TNF-α), disintegrin and metalloproteinase domain-containing protein 33 (ADAM33), interleukin-1 (IL1), interleukin-1 receptor antagonist (IL1RN), cystic fibrosis transmembrane conductance regulator (CFTR), and β_2-adrenergic receptor (ADRB2) are among the risk factors that contribute to the onset of COPD [5–7]. The development of COPD is contributed to by cellular senescence, inflammation, protease-antiprotease imbalance, epigenetic changes, oxidative stress, endoplasmic reticulum (ER) stress, mitochondrial dysfunction, advanced glycation end products, apoptosis, and cell death [8, 9]. COPD, which significantly affects the quality of life, negatively impacts societies economically and socially worldwide due to treatment costs and loss of workforce.

The endoplasmic reticulum (ER), which is part of the transport system in eukaryotic cells, is an organelle essential for cell survival [10]. The ER is the main location for lipid biosynthesis, calcium storage, and the synthesis of secretory or proteins associated with membranes and those directed to specific organelles and is vital for protein folding through specific chaperones and enzymes for newly made proteins [11]. Newly synthesized proteins cannot fold properly without undergoing various modifications. Most of the posttranslational modifications that ensure the proper folding of proteins' tertiary or quaternary structures (such as N-glycosylation, disulfide bond formation, hydroxylation, and oligomerization) occur in the ER [12]. ER, which serves as a quality control center, contains molecules called chaperones that facilitate the correct folding of proteins, such as Glucose-regulated protein 78 (Grp78) and Heat Shock Protein 70 (HSP70) [13]. Properly folded proteins are transported to the Golgi apparatus, while conditions that disrupt redox regulation and calcium homeostasis increase in reactive oxygen species (ROS) and disruption of the ROS-antioxidant balance, glucose deprivation, hypoxia, mutations in secreted proteins, viral infections, increased protein translation, or decreased protein folding capacity can lead to the accumulation of unfolded or misfolded proteins. Unfolded protein response (UPR) occurs to restore homeostasis in the cell. This unfolded protein response is a protective mechanism crucial for alleviating ER stress and resolving functional disruption. UPR activates a series of events involving intracellular signaling pathways to promote cell survival [14, 15]. Based on the cellular response obtained from UPR functioning, decisions can be made, such as inhibition of protein synthesis, regulation of gene expression, or apoptosis due to unresolved ER stress. Ultimately, unrestrained protein aggregates can lead to apoptotic cell death [13, 16]. When homeostatic balance cannot be restored as a result of this life-or-death decision, ER stress can contribute to the development of metabolic disorders, neurodegenerative disorders, cardiovascular diseases, and inflammatory lung diseases, including COPD [17].

This section provides an in-depth exploration of the role of ER stress in COPD, emphasizing the intricate relationship between ER stress response and inflammation. It also delves into the mechanisms underlying various cellular processes activated by the UPR, with a particular focus on the key ER stress triggers contributing to the pathogenesis of COPD.

2. The cell's life-or-death struggle under ER stress: The unfolded protein response

Predicting, responding to, and mitigating stress during metabolic regulation in the cell is crucial for maintaining homeostatic control. In a state of proteostatic balance, binding immunoglobulin proteins (BiPs) keep the stress transducer proteins, such as inositol-requiring enzyme 1 (IRE1), protein kinase RNA-like ER kinase (PERK), and activating transcription factor 6 (ATF6) in an inactive state. During ER stress, which can be caused by endogenous or exogenous sources, BiP binds with high affinity to misfolded or unfolded proteins. BiP dissociates from IRE1, PERK, and ATF6, thereby activating the UPR pathway. These activated three stress transducers (IRE1, PERK, and ATF6) stimulate target gene expression to restore cellular proteostasis and cell viability [13, 18, 19]. To mitigate ER stress, the response is first regulated by reducing the translocation of proteins to the ER through temporary adaptation, inducing the UPR, and finally triggering the apoptosis process if homeostatic balance cannot be restored [20].

2.1 UPR signaling pathways

2.1.1 IRE1-dependent unfolded protein response signaling pathway

Inositol-requiring enzyme 1, a type-I transmembrane protein involved in multiple cellular processes, has a serine/threonine kinase domain and an endoribonuclease (RNase) domain in C-terminal cytoplasmic region and an ER luminal domain in N-terminal [21, 22]. In humans, IRE1 exists in two isoforms: IRE1α and IRE1β. IRE1α is expressed broadly, while IRE1β is found abundantly only in intestinal and pulmonary epithelial and mucosal tissues [15, 23]. In the cellular response to ER stress, IRE1α acts as an early responder and immediately oligomerizes upon dissociation from BiP. This leads to autophosphorylation of its kinase domain, which, in turn, activates the endonuclease domain. With IRE1 activation, X-box binding protein 1 (XBP-1) mRNA is cleaved to produce the functionally active XBP-1 isoform (XBP1s) (**Figure 1**) [24, 25]. The XBP1s proteins, generated from the spliced mRNA, then translocate to the nucleus. To maintain ER homeostasis, the activated XBP1s isoform stimulates the transcription of target genes involved in essential ER protein folding chaperones, the transport and degradation pathways of unfolded or misfolded proteins *via* the ER-associated degradation (ERAD) and lipid biosynthesis [26]. In the ER, multiprotein complexes can detect, eliminate, ubiquitinate, and transport misfolded proteins to the 26S proteasome for degradation in the cytosol. This process is known as ERAD [27, 28]. If ER stress persists or becomes excessively severe, the UPR triggers apoptosis to eliminate the damaged cells [29]. Another degradation process, regulated IRE1-dependent decay (RIDD), can induce the degradation of an mRNA encoding ER-targeted proteins by active IRE1α. RIDD cleaves mRNAs coding for ER stress proteins, and prolonged activation of RIDD can lead the cell toward apoptosis [30, 31].

Inositol-requiring enzyme 1 also triggers different downstream signals and activates various functional cellular pathways by interacting with modulatory proteins, such as Heat Shock Protein (HSP), RING Finger Protein 13 (RNF13), and Poly (ADP-ribose) Polymerase 16 (PARP16) [30]. When homeostasis cannot be maintained against ER stress for an extended period, IRE1α interacts with tumor necrosis factor (TNF) receptor-associated factor 2 (TRAF2) and apoptosis signal-regulating kinase 1 (ASK1). The IRE1α-TRAF2-ASK1 complex can activate c-Jun N-terminal kinase (JNK)

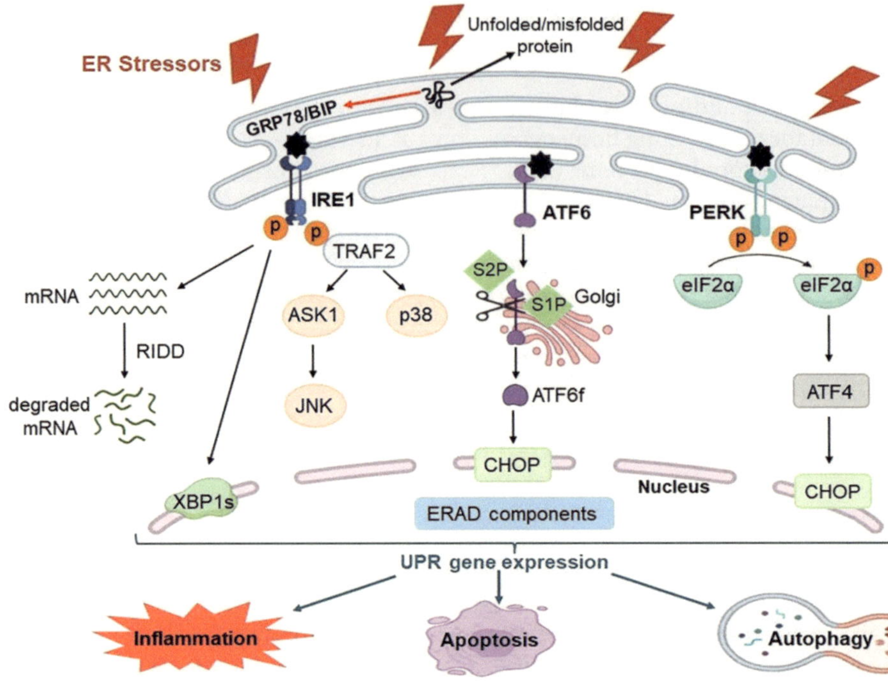

Figure 1.
UPR signaling pathways. ER stress, triggered by either internal or external factors, prompts BiP to strongly bind to misfolded or unfolded proteins. As a result, BiP detaches from IRE1, PERK, and ATF6, activating the UPR pathway. Once activated, these three stress sensors (IRE1, PERK, ATF6) drive the expression of target genes to reestablish cellular proteostasis and ensure cell survival.

and p38 mitogen-activated protein kinase-mediated signaling pathways, thereby triggering apoptosis [32].

2.1.2 ATF6-dependent unfolded protein response signaling pathway

Activating transcription factor 6 (ATF6) is synthesized as a type II ER transmembrane protein in all cell types and is expressed as two homologous regulatory proteins, ATF6α and ATF6β, which bind to ER stress response elements (ERSE) [15, 33]. On the cytoplasmic N-terminal side, it has a basic leucine zipper (bZIP) transcriptional activation domain [34]. Under normal conditions, ATF6 is localized to the ER membrane bound to BiP, but in conditions of ER stress due to the accumulation of unfolded proteins, ATF6α dissociates from BiP and is transported to the Golgi complex [26, 35]. During the unfolded protein response, ATF6, which enhances the functional capacity of the ER, is processed by two proteases after it reaches the Golgi. One of these proteases, serine protease site-1, cleaves ATF6 at its luminal domain, while the other, metalloprotease site-2, cleaves it at its N-terminal domain (**Figure 1**). Thus, the amino-terminal cytoplasmic fragment (ATF6f), which has the capacity to control transcription, is released [16, 36]. ATF6f, which enters the nucleus, binds to the ATF/cAMP response element (CRE) and ERSE, activating the expression of ER response proteins, such as BIP/GRP78, glucose-regulated protein 94 (GRP94), and C/EBP homolog protein (CHOP), thereby contributing to the maintenance of increased ER stress homeostasis [37–39]. In ER stress-mediated cell death, mitochondrial apoptotic pathways lead to the initiation of autophagy [40]. In addition, in mammals, ATF4 and ATF6 interact with the 26S proteasome to induce the HERP/Mif1 membrane protein, thus effectively allowing ERAD [41]. Moreover, CHOP plays a critical role in ER stress-induced alveolar epithelial cell aging and pulmonary fibrosis by activating the nuclear factor-kappa B pathway [42].

2.1.3 PERK-dependent unfolded protein response signaling pathway

Protein kinase RNA-like ER kinase, which has serine/threonine kinase activity, undergoes conformational changes by dissociating from BiP upon binding to unfolded proteins under ER stress conditions. After dissociation, PERK gains catalytic activity through oligomerization and autophosphorylation [43]. Active PERK facilitates the downregulation of translation by phosphorylating eukaryotic initiation factor 2α (eIF2α), thereby inhibiting protein synthesis. The reduced protein synthesis allows for the alleviation of the protein load in the ER [44, 45].

Moreover, the phosphorylation of eIF2α triggers an increase in the translation of particular mRNAs containing upstream open reading frames, which subsequently leads to a targeted rise in the cap-independent translation of ATF4 (**Figure 1**) [43, 46]. ATF4 is a transcriptional regulator of target genes involved in ER stress homeostasis, apoptosis, and oxidative stress homeostasis in response to cellular stress conditions such as hypoxic conditions and increased oxidative stress, in addition to ER stress. It is also known to be among the most pro-survival transmembrane ER proteins [47, 48]. Under persistent stress conditions, ATF4 heterodimerizes with CHOP (also known as DNA damage-inducible transcript 3; DDIT3) to induce apoptosis through their increased expression [48].

Under prolonged exposure to a specific stress source, the integrated stress response (ISR) is activated, and through ATF4, activating transcription factor 5 (ATF5), and CHOP, it increases the expression of ER target genes (chaperones, proteases, etc.) to mitigate the stress. If the chronic stress cannot be managed, this process then promotes the cell to undergo apoptosis [49].

3. ER stress triggers associated with COPD

In COPD pathogenesis, various inhaled triggers have the capacity to induce ER stress. Some of these include cigarette smoking, occupational and environmental exposure, disruptions in the antioxidant-oxidant balance, hypoxia, cell senescence, and genetic disorders (**Figure 2**) [50].

3.1 Cigarette smoking-mediated ER stress in COPD

Although many internal and external environmental factors have been identified in the development of COPD, cigarette smoking (CS) remains one of the highest risk factors (**Figure 2**) [51]. Considering that approximately one-fifth of the world's population smokes, it is not surprising that smoking is regarded as the highest contributing factor to the onset of lung diseases [52]. Tobacco products contain metals such as Cd, Pb, Ni, and Al; polycyclic aromatic hydrocarbons (PAHs) and other aromatic hydrocarbons such as benzene, toluene, and benzo(a)pyrene; nitrogenous compounds such as acetonitrile, benzonitrile, and 4-(methylnitrosamino)-1-(3-pyridyl)-1-butanone; aliphatic and unsaturated hydrocarbons such as isoprene, limonene, and ethylene;

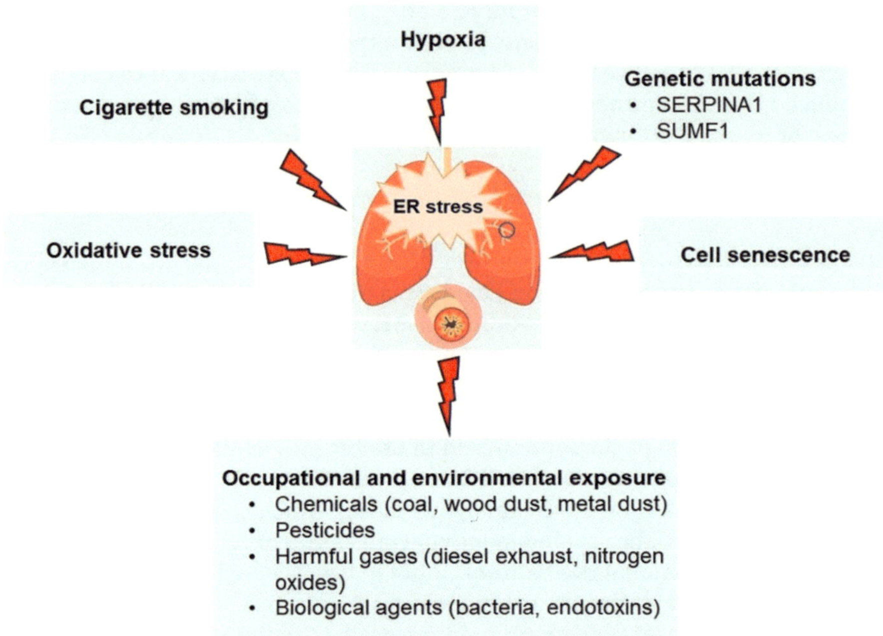

Figure 2.
ER stress triggers in COPD. ER stress triggers in COPD include cigarette smoking, occupational and environmental exposure, disruptions in the antioxidant-oxidant balance, hypoxia, cell senescence, and genetic disorders.

many aldehydes and ketones such as formaldehyde and 2,3-butanedione; alcohols and phenolic compounds such as glycerol, p-cresol, and 2-methoxy-4-methylphenol. In addition to all these harmful components, it also contains acids, anionic, cationic compounds, and gases, such as acetic acid, Cl^-, K^+, NO_3, CO, HCN, and NO [52, 53]. In lung tissue, CS induces inflammation and oxidative stress through increased reactive oxygen species (ROS) and reactive nitrogen species (RNS). As a result of chronic exposure to such harmful chemicals, airway epithelial cells undergo chronic inflammation and irreversible systemic oxidative stress, which can result in harm to cellular components like DNA or proteins, ultimately causing ER stress due to an insufficient antioxidant balance [54, 55]. In COPD, macrophages, neutrophils, and lymphocytes, including Tc1, Th1, Th17, and ILC3 cells, increase in the peripheral airways, lung parenchyma, and vascular area [56, 57]. Airway epithelial cells, fibroblasts, and endothelial cells produce mediators such as IL-8, leukotriene B4, and TNF-α, which sustain and amplify inflammation and contribute to oxidative stress [58]. Chronic ROS-mediated ER stress can activate various signaling pathways, leading to apoptosis and pyroptosis. IRE1α-XBP-1 and stimulator of interferon genes-TANK-binding kinase-1-interferon regulatory factor-3 (STING-TBK1-IRF3) pathways, activated by CS mediated ER stress, facilitate inflammasome formation through increased expression of NLR family pyrin domain-containing 3 (NLRP3) and proIL-1β. This activates caspase-1, which can exacerbate pyroptosis, cell death, and increased cytokine release, thereby intensifying damage to lung tissue [59].

Cigarette smoking contributes to the formation of ER stress by oxidizing protein-disulfide isomerase (PDI), an ER chaperone, thus triggering subsequent steps in the stress response [60]. By increasing oxidative stress, CS can damage proteins in lung tissue, leading to impaired cellular proteostasis and accumulation of misfolded proteins due to reduced proteasomal degradation in the alveolar epithelium. Consequently, the unresolved ER stress leads to the activation of apoptosis [61, 62].

3.2 Occupational and environmental exposure-mediated ER stress in COPD

Exposure to chemicals such as coal, wood dust, metal dust and fumes, pesticides, harmful gases such as diesel exhaust and nitrogen oxides, and biological agents such as mold, bacteria, or endotoxins can lead to COPD [63]. Exposure to particulate matter (PM 2.5; particles smaller than 2.5 μm in size) can activate the UPR pathway in response to PERK/eIF2α-mediated ER stress [64]. Increased ER stress and phosphorylation of eIF2α can induce the translation of mRNAs involved in protein synthesis, oxidative stress-antioxidant mechanisms, and apoptosis pathways. Chronic and systematic ER stress can induce apoptosis through CHOP [20, 65].

Environmental Pb exposure induces superoxide dismutase 1 (SOD1) expression, increases cleaved caspase-3 expression, and enhances the autophagy marker sequestosome 1 (p62/SQSTM1). The increased p62/SQSTM1 due to Pb exposure reflects oxidative stress, apoptosis, and autophagy dysfunction in the tissue [66]. In a study conducted to identify intracellular stress signaling pathways *in vivo* and *ex vivo*, it has been reported that PM 2.5 exposure leads to increased ROS production, phosphorylation of eIF2a, and an increase in ER stress-mediated CHOP expression. In response to ER stress, IRE1α is activated, inhibiting its activity in the addition of Xbp1 mRNA. The increased expression of CHOP induces PERK-mediated apoptosis [67]. Changes in human A549 and rat primary isolated alveolar type II cells exposed to asbestos have been investigated. This study revealed that exposure to asbestos leads to an elevation in the levels of IRE1 and XBP-1 in alveolar epithelial cells. The increase in ER stress proteins due to asbestos indicates an ER stress response, and the elevated ER stress also induces Ca^{2+} release, which triggers apoptosis [68].

Viruses utilize ER functions to replicate and can induce, modulate, or manipulate the UPR. They can also downregulate IRE1 to suppress the UPR. Bacteria that replicate within the ER, encountering a similar environment, can also induce and modulate the UPR [69]. Pathogens associated with respiratory diseases cause the induction of the UPR as part of the host ER stress response.

Legionella pneumophila, a respiratory pathogen, plays a role in mitochondrial gene expression, oxidative phosphorylation, mitochondrial fission and fusion, unfolded protein response pathways, chaperones, and the regulation of the apoptotic signaling pathway. By inducing the mitochondrial stress response, *Legionella pneumophila* upregulates UPR proteins, independently upregulates stress-related proteins, selectively induces ATF3, and suppresses the translation of ATF4 and CHOP [70]. *Legionella pneumophila* selectively activates ATF6 without inducing other UPR signaling pathways, initiating its translocation and the transcription of target genes [71]. *Pseudomonas aeruginosa* induces ER stress in bronchial epithelial cells by upregulating CHOP, GRP78, and growth arrest and DNA damage-inducible protein 34 (GADD34) expressions and triggers the integrated stress response (ISR) independently of ER stress. The ER stress response to *P. aeruginosa* in bronchial epithelial cells is induced *via* the TGF-β activated kinase-1-p38 mitogen-activated protein kinase (TAK1-p38 MAPK) pathway [72].

The bacterial community found in the lungs of patients with severe COPD has been found to be different from that in the lungs of control subjects and cystic fibrosis patients, specifically differing from the *Proteobacteria* or *Firmicutes phylum* [73].

Exposure to copper leads to an increase in the *Bacteroidaceae* family due to immune system disruption and microbial changes. The abundance of *Bacteroidaceae* is positively correlated with tissue ER stress and apoptosis proteins (GRP78, GRP94, eIF2α, ATF6, XBP1, CHOP) [74].

3.3 Genetic-mediated ER stress in COPD

α-1 antitrypsin (AAT) deficiency is due to mutations in the SERPINA1 gene, which is situated on chromosome 14 (14q32.1). This gene encodes the protein AAT, which protects tissues, especially in the lungs, from enzyme damage [75]. The most common alleles of the SERPINA1 gene are M, S, and Z. The M allele generates typical levels of AAT. S allele results in moderately reduced levels of AAT (approximately 60% of normal). Z allele is the most common mutation associated with AAT deficiency and results in significantly reduced levels of AAT (10–15% of normal) [76]. *MZ genotype* is usually asymptomatic but at increased risk for lung disease, especially if exposed to environmental risk factors like smoking. *SZ genotype* is moderately reduced AAT levels and increased risk for lung disease, particularly with smoking or other environmental factors. *ZZ genotype* is severely reduced AAT levels, a high risk for developing lung disease [77, 78]. In the Z allele, the substitution of a single amino acid (glutamic acid to lysine at position 342, or Glu342Lys) leads to abnormal folding of the AAT protein. The deficiency in circulating AAT results in decreased protection of lung tissue from neutrophil elastase, an enzyme that can degrade elastin and other structural proteins in the lungs [79].

The mutations in the Z variant of AAT deficiency can accelerate misfolding and lead to the formation of protein aggregates, contributing to lung disease. Increased neutrophil elastase activity has various effects that result in inflammation and a higher production rate of reactive oxygen species [80]. The aggregation of misfolded AAT proteins in the ER creates an overload of unfolded or misfolded proteins, leading to ER stress. The ER stress triggers the UPR, a cellular mechanism designed to alleviate the load of misfolded proteins and restore proper ER function [79, 81]. The COPD model generated in transgenic human Z-AT cells in response to cigarette smoke leads to intracellular polymerization through oxidation in pulmonary epithelial cells and results in increased expression of protein genes (with upregulation of PERK mRNA and ATF-4 mRNA) due to cellular inflammation and ER stress, as well as excessive cytokine release [82].

Another known genetic factor effective in COPD is mutations in sulfatase modifying factor 1 (SUMF1), which leads to the accumulation of excessively sulfated glycosaminoglycans (GAGs) in the lungs. In COPD patients, SUMF1 mRNA is relatively more abundant in lung tissue compared to its expression levels in other tissues. In COPD patients, splice variant 3 is expressed at the highest levels in lung tissue compared to all other examined tissues [83, 84].

3.4 Hypoxia-mediated ER stress in COPD

As a result of impaired lung function, hypoxia, hypoxemia, and hypercapnia can develop. The resulting hypoxia can lead to endothelial dysfunction due to the imbalance between vasodilation and vasoconstriction [85]. Hypoxia-inducible factor 1α (HIF-1α) is a transcription factor that responds to decreased cellular oxygen levels. In the lungs of COPD patients who smoke, the expression of HIF-1α increases due to heightened hypoxia, ROS, and systemic inflammation [86, 87]. Increased mitochondrial ROS triggers the inflammatory process through the activation of HIF-1, NF-κB, and pro-inflammatory cytokines, as well as inflammatory caspases, such as caspase-1 and caspase-12 [88]. The ROS response indirectly induces the activation of proteins involved in upstream autophagy signaling pathways, such as Jun-N-terminal kinase (JNK) and p38 mitogen-activated protein kinase (MAPK) [58]. Numerous studies in the literature indicate that hypoxic environments are crucial in the processes of tumor development, progression, and metastasis [89–91]. Under prolonged hypoxic conditions, the accumulation of misfolded or unfolded proteins leads to the activation of the UPR pathway, along with ER stress. The separation of the ER chaperone BIP activates the PERK pathway. Activated PERK phosphorylates eIF2, which upregulates the translation of ER stress response proteins, such as ATF4. In response to chronic ER stress, CHOP/GAAD 153 can induce death receptor 5 (DR5), initiating apoptosis [92–94].

3.5 Cell senescence-mediated ER stress in COPD

Cellular senescence is the cessation of the cell cycle as part of normal development, but it can also occur in response to stressors during the life cycle. By halting cell growth, it prevents the proliferation of old or unfit cells, serving as a defense process to protect the organism from potential dangers [95]. The process of cellular senescence can occur through the activation of tumor suppressor p53 *via* the replicative senescence pathway, or through the activation of cyclin-dependent kinase inhibitor p16INK4 in response to stress, leading to the inhibition of cyclin-dependent kinase-2/4. Ultimately, this results in the activation of cyclin-dependent kinase inhibitor p21CIP1, which causes cell cycle arrest [96, 97]. The process of cellular senescence is thought to be a driving force in chronic lung diseases such as COPD. In COPD, markers of cellular senescence, such as p16INK4a, p21CIP1, and senescence-associated β-galactosidase (SA-β-gal), are often elevated in lung tissues [98]. In COPD models, exposure to cigarette smoke in mouse and human lung epithelial cells induces cellular senescence through the activation of the p21-poly(ADP-ribose) polymerase (PARP)-1 pathway and upregulation of p21 [99, 100].

4. Conclusions and perspectives

This section examines the role of ER stress in COPD, focusing on its connection to inflammation, the mechanisms of UPR-triggered cellular processes, and the main ER stress triggers in the disease. The topics presented are extensively corroborated by a wealth of studies in the literature, underscoring their significance in the field. Research targeting therapeutic interventions and novel mediators linked to ROS, ER proteostasis, UPR signaling pathways, and cellular senescence—key contributors to COPD pathogenesis—holds substantial promise for advancing COPD treatment strategies.

Conflict of interest

The author declares no conflicts of interest.

Author details

Tugba Raika Kıran
Medical Biochemistry Department, Faculty of Medicine, Malatya Turgut Ozal University, Malatya, Turkey

*Address all correspondence to: raika.kiran@ozal.edu.tr

References

[1] Rodrigues SO, Cunha CMC, Soares GMV, Silva PL, Silva AR, Gonçalves-de-Albuquerque CF. Mechanisms, pathophysiology and currently proposed treatments of chronic obstructive pulmonary disease. Pharmaceuticals. 2021;**14**(10):979

[2] Labaki WW, Rosenberg SR. Chronic obstructive pulmonary disease. Annals of Internal Medicine. 2020;**173**(3):ITC17-ITC32

[3] Paleologos KE, Selim MYE, AMO M. Indoor air quality: Pollutants, health effects, and regulations. In: AMO M, Paleologos KE, Howari FM, editors. Pollution Assessment for Sustainable Practices in Applied Sciences and Engineering. Oxford: Butterworth-Heinemann; 2021. pp. 405-489

[4] Yang IA, Jenkins CR, Salvi SS. Chronic obstructive pulmonary disease in never-smokers: Risk factors, pathogenesis, and implications for prevention and treatment. The Lancet Respiratory Medicine. 2022;**10**(5):497-511

[5] Sandford AJ, Joos L, Paré PD. Genetic risk factors for chronic obstructive pulmonary disease. Current Opinion in Pulmonary Medicine. 2002;**8**(2):87-94

[6] Yuan C, Chang D, Lu G, Deng X. Genetic polymorphism and chronic obstructive pulmonary disease. International Journal of COPD. 2017;**12**:1385-1393

[7] Wu X, Yuan B, Lopez E, Bai C, Wang X. Gene polymorphisms and chronic obstructive pulmonary disease. Journal of Cellular and Molecular Medicine. 2014;**18**(1):15-26

[8] Choudhury G, MacNee W. Role of inflammation and oxidative stress in the pathology of ageing in COPD: Potential therapeutic interventions. COPD: Journal of Chronic Obstructive Pulmonary Disease. 2017;**14**(1):122-135

[9] Bezerra FS, Lanzetti M, Nesi RT, Nagato AC, Silva CP, Kennedy-Feitosa E, et al. Oxidative stress and inflammation in acute and chronic lung injuries. Antioxidants. 2023;**12**:548

[10] Yoshida H. ER stress and diseases. FEBS Journal. 2007;**274**(3):630-658

[11] Gorman AM, Healy SJM, Jäger R, Samali A. Stress management at the ER: Regulators of ER stress-induced apoptosis. Pharmacology & Therapeutics. 2012;**134**:306-316

[12] Arnold SM, Kaufman RJ. Protein synthesis, folding, modification, and secretion in mammalian cells. New Comprehensive Biochemistry. 2003;**38**:411-432

[13] Chen X, Shi C, He M, Xiong S, Xia X. Endoplasmic reticulum stress: Molecular mechanism and therapeutic targets. Signal Transduction and Targeted Therapy. 2023;**8**:352

[14] Dandekar A, Mendez R, Zhang K. Cross talk between ER stress, oxidative stress, and inflammation in health and disease. Methods in Molecular Biology. 2015;**1292**:205-214

[15] Li A, Song N-J, Riesenberg BP, Li Z. The emerging roles of endoplasmic reticulum stress in balancing immunity and tolerance in health and diseases: Mechanisms and opportunities. Frontiers in Immunology. 2020;**10**:3154

[16] Walter P, Ron D. The unfolded protein response: From stress pathway

to homeostatic regulation. Science. 2011;**334**:1081-1086

[17] Chipurupalli S, Samavedam U, Robinson N. Crosstalk between ER stress, autophagy and inflammation. Frontiers in Medicine. 2021;**8**:758311

[18] Oakes SA, Papa FR. The role of endoplasmic reticulum stress in human pathology. Annual Review of Pathology. 2015;**10**:173-119

[19] Chen X, Cubillos-Ruiz JR. Endoplasmic reticulum stress signals in the tumour and its microenvironment. Nature Reviews. 2021;**21**:72-88

[20] Ron D, Walter P. Signal integration in the endoplasmic reticulum unfolded protein response. Nature Reviews. Molecular Cell Biology. 2007;**8**:519-529

[21] Pan T, Zhang L, Miao K, Wang Y. A crucial role of endoplasmic reticulum stress in cellular responses during pulmonary arterial hypertension. American Journal of Translational Research. 2020;**12**(5):1481-1490

[22] Poothong J, Sopha P, Kaufman RJ, Tirasophon W. Domain compatibility in Ire1 kinase is critical for the unfolded protein response. FEBS Letters. 2010;**584**:3203-3208

[23] Yu Y, Yang A, Yu G, Wang H. Endoplasmic reticulum stress in chronic obstructive pulmonary disease: Mechanisms and future perspectives. Biomolecules. 2022;**12**:1637

[24] Yoshida H, Matsui T, Yamamoto A, Okada T, Mori K. XBP1 mRNA is induced by ATF6 and spliced by IRE1 in response to ER stress to produce a highly active transcription factor. Cell. 2001;**107**:881-891

[25] Calfon M, Zeng H, Urano F, Till JH, Hubbard SR, Harding HP, et al. IRE1 couples endoplasmic reticulum load to secretory capacity by processing the XBP-1 mRNA. Nature. 2002;**415**:92-96

[26] Park SM, Kang TI, So JS. Roles of XBP1s in transcriptional regulation of target genes. Biomedicine. 2021;**9**:791

[27] Needham PG, Guerriero CJ, Brodsky JL. Chaperoning endoplasmic reticulum–associated degradation (ERAD) and protein conformational diseases. Cold Spring Harbor Perspectives in Biology. 2019;**11**:a033928

[28] Lemus L, Goder V. Regulation of endoplasmic reticulum-associated protein degradation (ERAD) by ubiquitin. Cells. 2014;**3**:824-847

[29] Madden E, Logue SE, Healy SJ, Manie S, Samali A. The role of the unfolded protein response in cancer progression: From oncogenesis to chemoresistance. Biology of the Cell. 2019;**111**:1-17

[30] Wu J, He GT, Zhang WJ, Xu J, Huang QB. IRE1α signaling pathways involved in mammalian cell fate determination. Cellular Physiology and Biochemistry. 2016;**38**:847-858

[31] Pluquet O, Dejeans N, Bouchecareilh M, Lhomond S, Pineau R, Higa A, et al. Posttranscriptional regulation of PER1 underlies the oncogenic function of IRE alpha. Cancer Research. 2013;**73**:4732-4743

[32] Nishitoh H, Matsuzawa A, Tobiume K, Saegusa K, Takeda K, Inoue K, et al. ASK1 is essential for endoplasmic reticulum stress-induced neuronal cell death triggered by expanded polyglutamine repeats. Genes & Development. 2002;**16**(11):1345-1355

[33] Thuerauf DJ, Marcinko M, Belmont PJ, Glembotski CC. Effects

of the isoform-specific characteristics of ATF6 alpha and ATF6 beta on endoplasmic reticulum stress response gene expression and cell viability. The Journal of Biological Chemistry. 2007;**282**:22865-22878

[34] Kroeger H, Grimsey N, Paxman R, Chiang W-C, Plate L, Jones Y, et al. The unfolded protein response regulator ATF6 promotes mesodermal differentiation. Science Signaling. 2018;**11**(517):eaan5785

[35] Yamamoto K, Sato T, Matsui T, Sato M, Okada T, Yoshida H, et al. Transcriptional induction of mammalian ER quality control proteins is mediated by single or combined action of ATF6 alpha and XBP1. Developmental Cell. 2007;**13**:365-376

[36] Schroder M, Kaufman RJ. ER stress and the unfolded protein response. Mutation Research. 2005;**569**:29-63

[37] Urra H, Dufey E, Lisbona F, Rojas-Rivera D, Hetz C. When ER stress reaches a dead end. Biochimica et Biophysica Acta. 2013;**1833**:3507-3517

[38] Yang H, Niemeijer M, van de Water B, Beltma JB. ATF6 is a critical determinant of CHOP dynamics during the unfolded protein response. iScience. 2020;**23**(2):100860

[39] Shen J, Snapp EL, Lippincott-Schwartz J, Prywes R. Stable binding of ATF6 to BiP in the endoplasmic reticulum stress response. Molecular and Cellular Biology. 2005;**25**(3):921-932

[40] Kara M, Oztaş E. Endoplasmic reticulum stress-mediated cell death. In: Gali-Muhtasib H, Rahal ON, editors. Programmed Cell Death. London: InTech; 2020. pp. 51-65

[41] Read A, Schröder M. The unfolded protein response: An overview. Biology (Basel). 2021;**10**(5):384

[42] Jing X, Sun W, Yang X, Huang H, Wang P, Luo Q, et al. CCAAT/enhancer-binding protein (C/EBP) homologous protein promotes alveolar epithelial cell senescence via the nuclear factor-kappa B pathway in pulmonary fibrosis. The International Journal of Biochemistry & Cell Biology. 2022;**143**:106142

[43] Kadowaki H, Nishitoh H. Signaling pathways from the endoplasmic reticulum and their roles in disease. Genes (Basel). 2013;**4**(3):306-333

[44] Chen Y, Brandizzi F. IRE1: ER stress sensor and cell fate executor. Trends in Cell Biology. 2013;**23**(11):547-555

[45] Fan Y, Simmen T. Mechanistic connections between endoplasmic reticulum (ER) redox control and mitochondrial metabolism. Cells. 2019;**8**(9):1071

[46] Lu PD, Harding HP, Ron D. Translation reinitiation at alternative open reading frames regulates gene expression in an integrated stress response. The Journal of Cell Biology. 2004;**167**(1):27-33

[47] Huang W, Gong Y, Yan L. ER stress, the unfolded protein response and osteoclastogenesis: A review. Biomolecules. 2023;**13**(7):1050

[48] Neill G, Masson GR. A stay of execution: ATF4 regulation and potential outcomes for the integrated stress response. Frontiers in Molecular Neuroscience. 2023;**16**:1112253

[49] Almeida LM, Pinho BR, Duchen MR, Oliveira JMA. The PERKs of mitochondria protection during stress: Insights for PERK modulation in neurodegenerative and metabolic diseases. Biological Reviews. 2022;**97**:1737-1748

[50] Cloots E, Simpson MS, De Nolf C, Lencer WI, Janssens S, Grey MJ. Evolution and function of the epithelial cell-specific ER stress sensor IRE1β. Mucosal Immunology. 2021;**14**(6):1235-1246

[51] Yeap JW, Hyder-Ali IA, Ibrahim B, Tan ML. Chronic obstructive pulmonary disease and emerging ER stress-related therapeutic targets. Pulmonary Pharmacology & Therapeutics. 2023;**81**:102218

[52] Soleimani F, Dobaradaran S, De-la-Torre GE, Schmidt TC, Saeedi R. Content of toxic components of cigarette, cigarette smoke vs cigarette butts: A comprehensive systematic review. Science of the Total Environment. 2022;**813**:152667

[53] Dobaradaran S, Schmidt TC, Lorenzo-Parodi N, Kaziur-Cegla W, Jochmann MA, Nabipour I, et al. Polycyclic aromatic hydrocarbons (PAHs) leachates from cigarette butts into water. Environmental Pollution. 2020;**259**:113916

[54] Racanelli AC, Choi AMK, Choi ME. Autophagy in chronic lung disease. Progress in Molecular Biology and Translational Science. 2020;**172**:135-156

[55] Kıran TR, Otlu O, Karabulut AB. Oxidative stress and antioxidants in health and disease. Journal of Laboratory Medicine. 2023;**47**(1):1-11

[56] Barnes PJ. Inflammatory mechanisms in patients with chronic obstructive pulmonary disease. The Journal of Allergy and Clinical Immunology. 2016;**138**(1):16-27

[57] Eapen MS, Myers S, Walters EH, Sohal SS. Airway inflammation in chronic obstructive pulmonary diseases: A true paradox. Expert Review of Respiratory Medicine. 2017;**11**(10):827-839

[58] Albano GD, Gagliardo RP, Montalbano AM, Profita M. Overview of the mechanisms of oxidative stress: Impact in inflammation of the airway diseases. Antioxidants. 2022;**11**:2237

[59] Ding H, Wu R. The role of SHP2 in advancing COPD: Insights into oxidative stress, endoplasmic reticulum stress, and pyroptosis. Alternative Therapies in Health and Medicine. 2024;**18**:AT10792

[60] Kenche H, Ye ZW, Vedagiri K, Richards DM, Gao XH, Tew KD, et al. Adverse outcomes associated with cigarette smoke radicals related to damage to protein-disulfide isomerase. The Journal of Biological Chemistry. 2016;**291**:4763-4778

[61] Somborac-Bacura A, van der Toorn M, Franciosi L, Slebos DJ, Zanic-Grubisic T, Bischoff R, et al. Cigarette smoke induces endoplasmic reticulum stress response and proteasomal dysfunction in human alveolar epithelial cells. Experimental Physiology. 2013;**98**:316-325

[62] Yamada Y, Tomaru U, Ishizu A, Ito T, Kiuchi T, Ono A, et al. Decreased proteasomal function accelerates cigarette smoke-induced pulmonary emphysema in mice. Laboratory Investigation. 2015;**95**(6):625-634

[63] Elonheimo HM, Mattila T, Andersen HR, Bocca B, Ruggieri F, Haverinen E, et al. Environmental substances associated with chronic obstructive pulmonary disease-a scoping review. International Journal of Environmental Research and Public Health. 2022;**19**:3945

[64] Schroder M, Kaufman RJ. The mammalian unfolded protein response. Annual Review of Biochemistry. 2005;**74**:739-789

[65] Zinszner H, Kuroda M, Wang X, Batchvarova N, Lightfoot RT, Remotti H, et al. CHOP is implicated in programmed cell death in response to impaired function of the endoplasmic reticulum. Genes & Development. 1998;**12**:982-995

[66] Corsetti G, Romano C, Stacchiotti A, Pasini E, Dioguardi FS. Endoplasmic reticulum stress and apoptosis triggered by sub-chronic lead exposure in mice spleen: A histopathological study. Biological Trace Element Research. 2016;**178**:86-97

[67] Laing S, Wang G, Briazova T, Zhang C, Wang A, Zheng Z, et al. Airborne particulate matter selectively activates endoplasmic reticulum stress response in the lung and liver tissues. American Journal of Physiology. Cell Physiology. 2010;**299**(4):C736-C749

[68] Kamp DW, Liu G, Cheresh P, Kim S-J, Mueller A, Lam AP, et al. Asbestos-induced alveolar epithelial cell apoptosis the role of endoplasmic reticulum stress response. American Journal of Respiratory Cell and Molecular Biology. 2013;**49**(6):892-901

[69] Celli J, Tsolis RM. Bacteria, the endoplasmic reticulum and the unfolded protein response: Friends or foes? Nature Reviews Microbiology. 2014;**13**(2):71-82

[70] Noack J-M, Jimenez-Morales D, Stevenson E, Moss T, Jang G, Krogan NJ, et al. Dynamic proteomics profiling of Legionella pneumophila infection unveils modulation of the host mitochondrial stress response pathway. SSRN Electronic Journal. 2020;**1**:e3631502

[71] Ibe NU, Subramanian A, Mukherjee S. Non-canonical activation of the ER stress sensor ATF6 by legionella pneumophila effectors. Life Science Alliance. 2021;**4**(12):1-16

[72] van't Wout EF, van Schadewijk A, van Boxtel R, Dalton LE, Clarke HJ, Tommassen J, et al. Virulence factors of pseudomonas aeruginosa induce both the unfolded protein and integrated stress responses in airway epithelial cells. PLoS Pathogens. 2015;**11**(6):e1004946

[73] Sze MA, Hogg JC, Sin DD. Bacterial microbiome of lungs in COPD. International Journal of COPD. 2014;**9**:229-238

[74] Ma F, Huo Y, Li H, Yang F, Liao J, Han Q, et al. New insights into the interaction between duodenal toxicity and microbiota disorder under copper exposure in chicken: Involving in endoplasmic reticulum stress and mitochondrial toxicity. Chemico-Biological Interactions. 2022;**366**:110132

[75] Hazaria YM, Bashira A, Habib M, Bashira S, Habibb H, Qasim MA, et al. Alpha-1-antitrypsin deficiency: Genetic variations, clinical manifestations and therapeutic interventions. Mutation Research. 2017;**773**:14-25

[76] Seixas S, Marque PI. Known mutations at the cause of alpha-1 antitrypsin deficiency an updated overview of SERPINA1 variation spectrum. The Application of Clinical Genetics. 2021;**14**:173-194

[77] Tzortzaki EG, Siafakas NM. Genetic susceptibility to chronic obstructive pulmonary disease. European Respiratory Monograph. 2006;**38**:84-99

[78] Strange C. Alpha-1 antitrypsin deficiency associated COPD. Clinics in Chest Medicine. 2020;**41**(3):339-345

[79] Karatas E, Bouchecareilh M. Alpha 1-antitrypsin deficiency: A disorder of proteostasis-mediated protein folding and trafficking pathways. International

Journal of Molecular Sciences. 2020;**21**(4):1493

[80] Greene CM, Marciniak SJ, Teckman J, Ferrarotti I, Brantly ML, Lomas DA, et al. α1-antitrypsin deficiency. Nature Reviews Disease Primers. 2016;**2**:16051

[81] Perlmutter DH. α1-antitrypsin deficiency: A misfolded secretory protein variant with unique effects on the endoplasmic reticulum. Endoplasmic Reticulum Stress Disease. 2016;**3**:63-72

[82] Alam S, Li Z, Atkinson C, Jonigk D, Janciauskiene S, Mahadeva R. Z a1-antitrypsin confers a proinflammatory phenotype that contributes to chronic obstructive pulmonary disease. American Journal of Respiratory and Critical Care Medicine. 2014;**189**(8):909-931

[83] Weidner J, Jarenbäck L, de Jong K, Vonk JM, van den Berge M, Brandsma CA, et al. Sulfatase modifying factor 1 (SUMF1) is associated with chronic obstructive pulmonary disease. Respiratory Research. 2017;**18**:77

[84] Jarenbäck L, Frantz S, Weidner J, Ankerst J, Nihlén U, Bjermer L, et al. Single-nucleotide polymorphisms in the sulfatase-modifying factor 1 gene are associated with lung function and COPD. ERJ Open Research. 2022;**8**(2):00668-02021

[85] Kent BD, Mitchell PD, McNicholas WT. Hypoxemia in patients with COPD: Cause, effects, and disease progression. International Journal of COPD. 2011;**6**:199-208

[86] Shukla HD, Walters EH, Simpson JL, Kelly S, Wark PAB, ROF O't, et al. Hypoxia-inducible factor and bacterial infections in chronicobstructive pulmonary disease. Respirology. 2020;**25**:53-63

[87] Sabit R, Thomas P, Shale DJ, Collins P, Linnane SJ. The effects of hypoxia on markers of coagulation and systemic inflammation in patients with COPD. Chest. 2010;**138**(1):47-51

[88] Nakano H, Nakajima A, Sakon-Komazawa S, Piao JH, Xue X, Okumura K. Reactive oxygen species mediate crosstalk between NF-kappaB and JNK. Cell Death and Differentiation. 2006;**13**:730-737

[89] Talks KL, Turley H, Gatter KC, Maxwell PH, Pugh CW, Ratcliffe PJ, et al. The expression and distribution of the hypoxia-inducible factors HIF-1α and HIF-2α in normal human tissues, cancers, and tumor-associated macrophages. The American Journal of Pathology. 2000;**157**:411-421

[90] Rohwer N, Lobitz S, Daskalow K, Jons T, Vieth M, Schlag PM, et al. HIF-1alpha determines the metastatic potential of gastric cancer cells. British Journal of Cancer. 2009;**100**:772-781

[91] Chipurupalli S, Kannan E, Tergaonkar V, D'Andrea R, Robinson N. Hypoxia induced ER stress response as an adaptive mechanism in cancer. International Journal of Molecular Sciences. 2019;**20**(3):749

[92] Harding HP, Zhang Y, Bertolotti A, Zeng H, Ron D. Perk is essential for translational regulation and cell survival during the unfolded protein response. Molecular Cell. 2000;**5**(5):897-904

[93] Bi M, Naczki C, Koritzinsky M, Fels D, Blais J, Hu N, et al. ER stress-regulated translation increases tolerance to extreme hypoxia and promotes tumor growth. The EMBO Journal. 2005;**24**:3470-3481

[94] He Q, Luo X, Jin W, Huang Y, Reddy MVR, Reddy EP, et al. Celecoxib

and a novel COX-2 inhibitor ON09310 upregulate death receptor 5 expression via GADD153/CHOP. Oncogene. 2008;**27**:2656-2660

[95] Herranz N, Gil J. Mechanisms and functions of cellular senescence. The Journal of Clinical Investigation. 2018;**128**(4):1238-1246

[96] Muñoz-Espín D, Serrano M. Cellular senescence: From physiology to pathology. Nature Reviews. Molecular Cell Biology. 2014;**15**:482-496

[97] Barnes PJ, Baker J, Donnelly LE. Cellular senescence as a mechanism and target in chronic lung diseases. American Journal of Respiratory and Critical Care Medicine. 2019;**200**(5):556-564

[98] Parikh P, Wicher S, Khandalavala K, Pabelick CM, Britt RD, Prakash YS. Cellular senescence in the lung across the age spectrum. Journal of Physiology Lung Cellular and Molecular Physiology. 2019;**316**:826-842

[99] Yao H, Sundar IK, Gorbunova V, Rahman I. P21-PARP-1 pathway is involved in cigarette smoke-induced lung DNA damage and cellular senescence. PLoS One. 2013;**8**(11):e80007

[100] Tsuji T, Aoshiba K, Nagai A. Cigarette smoke induces senescence inalveolar epithelial cells. American Journal of Respiratory Cell and Molecular Biology. 2004;**31**:643-649

Chapter 5

Online Respiratory Rehabilitation in Patients with COPD

Paula Irina Barata and Maria Daniela Mot

Abstract

Chronic obstructive pulmonary disease (COPD) is a common preventable and treatable disease characterized by persistent respiratory symptoms and airflow limitation caused by airway or alveolar abnormalities. With the advent of the pandemic, online respiratory rehabilitation for patients with COPD has become a major point of interest for both patients and doctors. Pulmonary rehabilitation is an integrative approach to achieve quality, accessibility, cost-effectiveness, and patient participation. Studies confirm that remotely supported RP with various telemedicine devices is not inferior to traditional RP. Most PR interventions could be delivered in primary care by adopting telemedicine solutions (e.g., via smartphone) and chronic care model to improve timely access, enrollment and engagement for COPD patients.

Keywords: COPD, digitalization of healthcare, pulmonary rehabilitation, respiratory disease, spirometry

1. Introduction

Chronic obstructive pulmonary disease represents one of the pathologies with the highest addressability in the emergency room and occupies a significant number of hospitalizations on our ward. In our country, due to the large number of smoking patients, it is estimated that approximately one million people suffer from this pathology, more than that, it has become the third cause of death in the world, thus surpassing pathologies such as hypertension and diabetes.

Due to the large number of patients with obstructive pulmonary disease, I chose to build my work around this pathology because every day both doctors and nurses are in the situation of caring for such a patient, which practically represents a challenge.

Another reason why I chose this topic is the fact that lately, we are no longer talking about a single disease, but it is important to redefine the phenotypes for personalizing the treatment of patients, which I will detail in the general part of the paper.

The most important thing is that recently, more and more doctors have chosen to introduce COPD patients to pulmonary rehabilitation programs, which has led to a significant increase in the quality of life of patients and if the COVID pandemic has brought many disasters worldwide in terms of as far as pulmonary rehabilitation is concerned, it has brought an extraordinary benefit by performing the exercises at a distance, that is, in the online environment. The patients were able to carry out their training inside their home through online platforms with the hospital's physiotherapists such as ZOOM or even already registered platforms such as the PNEUMOCONTROL application made by the specialists of the Victor Babeş hospital in Timişoara, a platform that can be enjoyed by the entire population.

Although at first, every doctor was perhaps reserved about this online approach to rehabilitation exercises, it later proved to be extremely successful with patients as they no longer had to travel to the hospital for a new program and could do it from inside their home, and more than that, the patients' feed-backs were extraordinarily good because they also had the support of their families, and then everything was much easier.

2. Online respiratory rehabilitation in patients with COPD

Chronic obstructive pulmonary disease is a real problem worldwide, being ranked as the third cause of death and occurring mostly in underdeveloped countries. By the year 2030, a decrease in premature deaths caused by non-communicable diseases such as chronic obstructive pulmonary disease is desired, but due to the increasing number of smokers, this is quite difficult to achieve [1]. Until 2019, we were talking about a number of more than 3 million people who died because of this pathology, a number that will increase progressively from 1 year to the next [2].

Like most lung pathologies, COPD is underdiagnosed both in Romania and in other European countries, patients tending to go to the medical service when they have an exacerbation and most of the time their lung function is already very low which leads to a well-known symptomatology marked, by dyspnea and fatigue accompanied by a chronic cough. Thus, we are surprised that at this moment the patients are already in stages III or IV on the GOLD scale.

In order to better understand this pathology, we must know that the term COPD was introduced in 1960, thus bringing together the two pathologies that are the basis of chronic obstructive pulmonary disease, namely chronic bronchitis and pulmonary emphysema. It is characterized by a chronic obstruction of the airways that is often incompletely reversible and with a high degree of progressivity, especially if the patient does not stop smoking or exposure to respiratory noxes and does not correctly follow the treatment recommended by the attending physician. It is also a pathology that in turn causes other comorbidities, making the status of this type of patient more and more difficult.

Regarding the way this disease occurs, it should be noted that smoking is the main cause of the disease, but of course, there are other causes that we will go over below.

- Smoking—first of all, we must know that in our brain, there is a nicotinic receptor that is stimulated by nicotine and thus the release of dopamine occurs, which gives people a feeling of pleasure and satisfaction when they light up a cigarette, but this does not last very long and the smoker will want to light up a cigarette again, and this interval will progressively decrease, and this leads to more and more cigarettes consumed per day. Smoking has been shown to kill more people than alcohol, traffic accidents, illegal drugs, obesity, suicide attempts, or murder combined. Passive smoking is also not to be neglected, and here we are talking about second-hand and third-hand smoking, with which ordinary people are not very familiar [3].

- Genetic factors—although it is not a fully elucidated subject, even if there are family and twin studies regarding this issue, we must still remember the deficiency of alpha 1 antitrypsin, coded by SERPINA1 genes, a 52kd glycoprotein that has the highest impact on neutrophil elastase (this being involved in the destruction of the alveolar wall).

- Age and sex—in terms of age, COPD is the prerogative of people over 50 with a significant history of smoking, and in terms of gender we can say that recently studies have shown an equal prevalence between the sexes. Age can also be an important risk factor because it has already been proven that even when a person is not a smoker, after the age of 35 they start to lose their lung function.

- Other factors—atmospheric pollution, nutrition, occupational exposure to noxes and gases, asthma and bronchial hyperactivity, infections.

The symptomatology of the patient with obstructive pulmonary disease is quite well defined and is more obvious at night and in the morning, although patients tend to neglect it for a long time, being already familiar with it and basing this aspect on smoking. But the most important symptoms that appear are marked by

- Cough with expectoration which can sometimes become muco-purulent when we talk about exacerbations and which most frequently occurs in the morning upon waking up and which can sometimes be in a much larger quantity than usual if there is a concomitant COPD-bronchiectasis, patients who are perfect candidates for pulmonary rehabilitation programs.

- Dyspnea is the second symptom that is perceived in the patient with COPD, being progressive and felt more and more once the patient shows significant decreases in Forced Expiratory Volume (FEV1). It is also important to quantify the dyspnea of our patients through scales such as Modified Medical Research Council (mMRC), BORG to be able to have a clearer picture of the patient.

- Wheezing, not always perceptible. When there is it is generated especially by quasi-permanent narrowing of the bronchial lumens, the presence of secretions, and often also bronchospasm.

- Chest pains, gastro-esophageal reflux; installation a pneumothorax through the rupture of an emphysematous bulla.

- Limited exercise capacity due to dyspnea, muscle dysfunction, and deconditioning.

- Symptoms related to the comorbidities and/or systemic effects of COPD.

The diagnosis of this pathology is not a very complicated one, and suspicion should be raised in all patients who have a history of smoking or occupational exposure accompanied by cough, dyspnea, morning expectoration, and of course these things being completed by a spirometry and a lung X-ray.

In some cases, chest pain may also occur due to increased pressure in the pulmonary artery—right angle or in the case of emphysema patients, a pneumothorax may occur due to the bursting of an emphysema bubble.

Returning to the two symptoms—cough and dyspnea, it is important to note that the first one is more frequent in the morning, it is mostly chronic and presents exacerbations in the cold season, it can change its character by becoming purulent, and a larger amount of sputum suggests most often an advancement of the disease toward the association of bronchiectasis. The installation of dyspnea most often starts to worry the patient because at this stage he can no longer carry out his daily activities normally, and compared to asthmatic patients, the dyspnea of the patient with COPD is persistent and progressive, being marked by the functional decline of FEV1. There are two highly used and beneficial scales that are used in the quantification of dyspnea, namely the mMRC and the BORG scale.

The mMRC presents five grades depending on the severity of the patient and is an extremely easy-to-use scale.

- Grade 0: dyspnea during intense physical exertion.
- Grade 1: dyspnea when walking fast or climbing a gentle slope.
- Grade 2: walking slower than people of the same age due to dyspnea, or the need to stop when climbing a floor at your own pace.
- Grade 3: forced to stop after less than 100 m of self-paced walking due to dyspnea.
- Grade 4: dyspnea too marked to be able to leave the house, or when performing routine activities such as washing or dressing.

Another clinical characteristic is represented by the frequently exacerbating patient in which the symptomatology is potentiated and most of the time this exacerbation occurs due to a viral or bacterial respiratory infection and usually these amplify three determinant factors for the cardiopulmonary risk contributing to the increased risk of events cardiac and pulmonary.

Another important point once the diagnosis of COPD has been established is its classification using the Global Initiative for Chronic Obstructive Lung Disease (GOLD) scale for a correct approach and correct treatment for the patient with COPD (**Table 1** and **Figure 1**) [2].

In patients with FEV1/FVC < 0.70		
GOLD 1	Easy	VEMS ≥80% as predicted
GOLD 2	Medium	50% ≤ VEMS <80% as predicted
GOLD 3	Severe	30% ≤ VEMS <50% as predicted
GOLD 4	Very severe	VEMS ≤30% as predicted
Adapted GOLD Guideline 2024 [2].		

Table 1.
Severity grades of COPD.

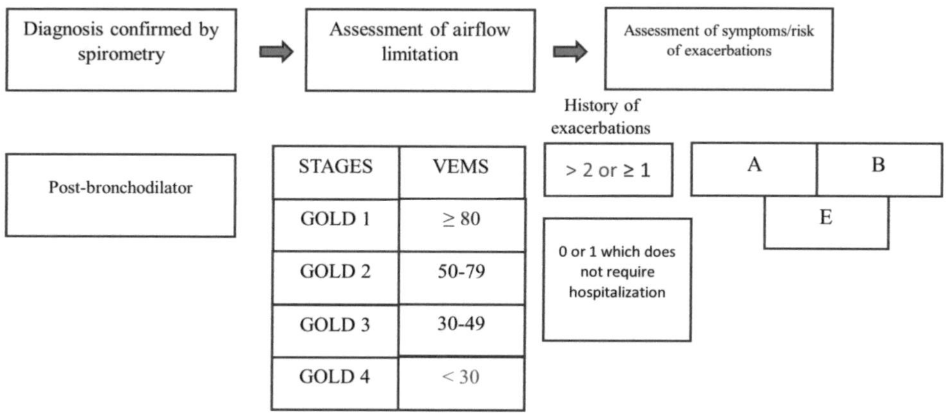

Figure 1.
COPD classification adapted according to the GOLD 2024 guideline [2].

Also the investigation of a patient with COPD is extremely important and we mention some of the most important investigations

- Functional explorations—spirometry is the GOLD standard in the diagnosis of COPD where we can observe an obstructive ventilatory dysfunction, the value of which does not change when taking a bronchodilator (FEV1 < 80%, FEV1/FVC < 0.7 of the predicted value), the factor of carbon monoxide transfer which assesses emphysematous damage and most importantly the 6-minute walk test which in clinical practice is often neglected but which brings valuable information about the patient. The 6-minute walk test (6MWT) measures the patient's maximum distance covered in 6 minutes. At the beginning and at the end of the test, the dynamics of the following parameters are evaluated: SaO2, AV, dyspnea according to the Borg scale and fatigue. In clinical practice, the 6MWT is important in evaluating prognosis, predicting mortality, and the effectiveness of certain therapies [2].

- Laboratory analysis—in the case of patients with hypercapnic respiratory failure, it is very beneficial to monitor the Pco2 value through an ASTRUP-type gasometry because they frequently show significant increases in carbon dioxide, decreases in oxygen, changes in blood Ph, but also increases in bicarbonate through a compensatory metabolic mechanism, polycythemia occurs in the context of chronic hypoxemia and may be an indicator of the need to institute long-term oxygen therapy, changes in eosinophils.

- EKG—may indicate right heart hypertrophy that precedes chronic pulmonary heart disease.

- Imaging—lung X-ray in the case of patients with COPD is not necessarily a helpful investigation in the early stages because most of the time this is normal, it can be useful in the case of exacerbations where it can present a pneumonic focus, or in advanced cases through bursting an emphysema bubble to visualize a pneumothorax or when hyperinflation, flattening of the diaphragm, and increased diameter of the pulmonary artery occur. CT is not a routine investigation, but it can be useful in some situations, namely the follow-up of emphysematous progression.

The treatment of patient with COPD is quite well-known, and here of course we are talking about correct management marked by the reduction of risk factors, hospitalizations, exacerbations, and appropriate pharmacological and non-pharmacological treatment. As for non-pharmacological treatment, it lends itself to lung volume resection surgery, lung transplantation, and respiratory rehabilitation.

Recently, respiratory rehabilitation has occupied an extremely important place in the pulmonology departments, and it should be emphasized that it is good to start as soon as possible, namely from stage II GOLD, and according to the definition of ATS, ERS, in fact, respiratory rehabilitation is a multidisciplinary condition including, in addition to classic exercises, psycho-social programs, elements of nutrition and diet, individual education programs with the help of online platforms. Most programs start from the hospital (in-patient program) and it is very important for the patient to continue at home for the desired results (out-patient program), and the duration of such a program is at least 2 months [2].

What is the role of a rehabilitation program in the case of a patient with COPD?

- Reduction of patient mortality and hospitalizations.
- Reduction of exacerbations and addressability to the on-call room, thus reducing the costs for such patients.
- Reducing symptoms and even improving them by decreasing the degree of dyspnea and improving the patient's cough.
- Reintegration into social and professional life.
- Improving the patient's quality of life through quality sleep, optimizing nutritional status.
- Increasing resistance to effort.

2.1 Indications and contraindications

The start of a pulmonary rehabilitation program can be done at any stage of the disease's evolution, whether we have a patient in the condition period, in exacerbation or a patient at home with the appropriate treatment. Although patients are still not very familiar with these programs recently, especially post-COVID, respiratory rehabilitation has started to gain more and more ground. So we have some indications that we should follow in our patients.

- Dyspnea at rest or on exertion (mMRC grade III) [4]
- Hypoxic or hypercapnic respiratory failure
- Reduced exercise tolerance
- Weight loss due to prolonged respiratory effort
- Significant degradation of symptoms

Contraindications in the case of a rehabilitation program can be absolute or relative; in the first category, we find the following pathologies.

- Severe pulmonary hypertension, recent myocardial infarction, angina pectoris
- Bone fractures
- Transmissible infectious pathology
- Mental illness, dementia
- Recent cerebrovascular accidents

2.2 Relative contraindications

- In some countries, smoking is a relative contraindication for starting a respiratory rehabilitation program
- Lack of motivation
- Severe anemia
- Progressive neuromuscular disease

At the same time, a rigorous evaluation of the patient through investigations that assume is also important.

- Rigorous patient history
- Biological balance
- Imaging investigations—radiography, chest CT
- Spirometry, dLCO, body-plethysmography
- EKG, cardiological consultation
- Body mass index analysis
- 6 MWT
- Certain quizzes—mMRC, BORG, STOP-BANG, CAT, and SGRQ

The 6-minute walk test is the cheapest screening method, and it measures the distance traveled by the patient on a linear route in 6 minutes. Blood pressure, peripheral oxygen saturation, body mass index, and distance covered are recorded. Using standard formulas, the predicted distance is calculated for the patient's age, gender, and height [5].

Online pulmonary rehabilitation actually involves several steps in addition to starting exercises to help the patient improve the two primary symptoms, namely the relief of dyspnea and cough. These online programs also include education in terms of lifestyle, nutrition, quitting smoking, self-management of symptoms, and oxygen therapy. For example, one such program offered by MorlenHealth brings to the fore respiratory rehabilitation programs that combine individual counseling with seminars and exercise classes, and like other programs, these last 12 weeks, and the results are visible.

In 2022 Paula Irina Barata et al. They conducted a study to see if online pulmonary rehabilitation can be as effective as in-patient respiratory rehabilitation and exercise with a physical therapist. This was desired because the pandemic forced us to find new solutions for our patients to continue the programs that had to be carried out by them. This study was based on the PneumoControl application (a medical information application) where there were all the patients who accessed this platform, and thus we divided them into two groups—those who were going to perform pulmonary rehabilitation online and those who performed the program in the ward ours for a period of 3 months. All those brought into the studio were evaluated in terms of lung volumes, 6-minute walk test, CAT questionnaire, Borg scale, test (mMRC). It was also taken into account that the patients were over 45 years old, without exacerbations in the last 3 months, without participation in a pulmonary rehabilitation program in the last 3 months, having a mobile phone for those who were in the online group and a pulse oximeter. Exclusion criteria: exacerbation in the last 3 months, other comorbidities that could interfere with their current health status, use of medications that could affect the response to exercise, active smoking status, musculoskeletal conditions that could affect exercise, a vision impairment that could affect the use of the mobile application, not having a stationary bike at home, a cognitive impairment that could affect the understanding of exercises. The duration of the program was 21 days, 5 days a week being led by a physiotherapist, and the patients at home were monitored through the mobile application (the feasibility of application was also demonstrated in other previous studies). Training sessions followed ATS recommendations, lasted 45–60 minutes, and consisted of diaphragmatic breathing exercises, pursed-lip breathing, and strength and endurance training. Thus, 72 patients were part of the group of those admitted to the hospital, respectively 58 of those enrolled online, and comparative studies were made before and after rehabilitation in each separate group, followed by the comparison of the data between the two groups. Following the 21 days of both physical and online pulmonary rehabilitation, significant increases in the CAT, BORG, and mMRC questionnaires and the increase in the 6-minute test distance were observed in both groups. Online pulmonary rehabilitation does not appear to be at all inferior to classical; moreover, online pulmonary rehabilitation demonstrated greater increases in the CAT score and increased distance in the 6-minute test compared to physical rehabilitation, which is probably explained by the fact that patients feel much quieter at home and perform rehabilitation exercises much more thoroughly.

Also, Bourne et al. demonstrated the same in a similar study in 2017 using the myMHealth platform, and it practically served as a springboard for subsequent studies in opening up this online rehabilitation opportunity [6]. However, an extremely important thing must be pointed out regarding pulmonary rehabilitation in Romania compared to other countries in Europe—because the national health system in our country only pays for 3 weeks for carrying out the programs compared to other countries where the programs are run over a period of 6–12 weeks so sometimes comparisons in our case can be deficient, but we can say that online pulmonary rehabilitation is extremely welcome for both patients and hospitals by decongesting the large number of people who turn to our service.

Skeletal muscle is also a key point in patients with lung disease, and exercises that improve its function should be emphasized because improvements in capillarization and increases in myoglobin levels may occur following rehabilitation.

However, telerehabilitation is not a very new method because there have been publications in this direction since 1998. However, since then, it has improved and advanced, existing both in the pulmonary, cardiac, and neurological fields.

It is also important to know that a study published in 2022 by MEGHAN RALEIGH et al. demonstrated through quality-of-life questionnaires that were similar in both in-hospital and online pulmonary rehabilitation patients that there were no significant differences in its role for patients [7].

During the years of the pandemic, we have observed that the benefits of online pulmonary rehabilitation are similar to hospital ones, as demonstrated in the articles above, and a considerable number of patients are more open to this type of rehabilitation, as some prefer the privacy of the home, others they simply reduce their costs in terms of an admission, and at home most have family support which has been shown to be another factor that positively influences patients' progress [8].

So we can say that, indeed, pharmacological therapy remains the standard in the treatment of COPD, but sometimes it can be insufficient in solving a case of COPD, and that is why supplementing the therapy with pulmonary rehabilitation either in the hospital or online is of great interest and this has been demonstrated since ancient times when Alvan Barach showed that dyspnea can be relieved by the posture—bent forward.

2.3 Components of pulmonary rehabilitation

There are a number of patients who may be in an acute phase of the disease and it is very important for them to start rehabilitation exercises as soon as possible, so telerehabilitation is a favorable solution for them (**Figure 2**). So that online respiratory rehabilitation can be considered a therapeutic method that has given favorable results; this has been demonstrated in countless studies, but it can also be a limitation of this method because some patients are not familiar with the technology and then cannot use such equipment [9].

> *"Pulmonary rehabilitation is a comprehensive intervention based on a thorough patient assessment followed by patient-tailored therapies that include but are not limited to, exercise training, education, and behavior change, designed to improve the physical and psychological condition of people with chronic respiratory disease and to promote the long-term adherence to health-enhancing behaviors" [10].*

So whether we introduce the patient to a rehabilitation program in the hospital or online, we must take into account certain assessments—risk factors such as smoking and sedentary lifestyle, assessment of comorbidities such as hypertension, diabetes, thyroid diseases, reflux gastro-esophageal, nutritional factors through BMI assessment, psychological assessment to detect depression or anxiety, sleep assessment is a point of maximum importance either through polygraphy or somnography, assessment of the quality of life through the SGRQ test.

Also, recently, studies have been done, and it has been shown that listening to music while performing rehabilitation exercises leads to better adherence to the program because patients feel more relaxed and happier and can more easily complete the rehabilitation program. Jun Okamoto et al. demonstrated in a study that

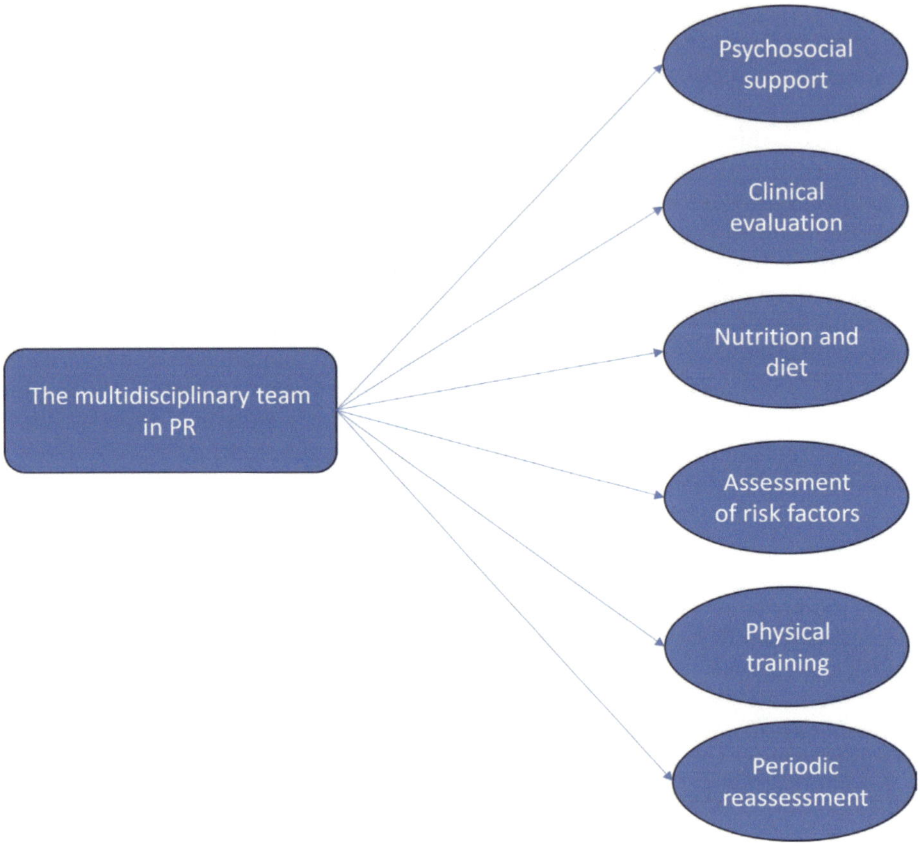

Figure 2.
Components of pulmonary rehabilitation.

music therapy has beneficial effects on COPD patients with dyspnea but did not show significant changes in depression and anxiety, which were expected to improve significantly, but there are still not enough studies in this direction. But I believe that online pulmonary rehabilitation and music therapy can have extremely good effects on patients [11]. Minghui Shi et al. have tried more than that, namely a combination of pulmonary telerehabilitation with music therapy and controlling the patient's breathing by singing—COPDMELODY, only that this combination has some shortcomings because it is quite difficult to control the patient at home, most studies of this kind doing- in the hospital [12].

3. Conclusions

Pulmonary rehabilitation addresses several lung pathologies that present airflow limitation, hyperinflation, hypoxemia, and hypercapnia, but COPD remains the pathology with the greatest addressability and the most convincing results so far, something proven in countless studies. The role of rehabilitation is very clear: it is aimed at increasing the quality of life, re-introducing the patient into the social environment, resuming the best quality of daily activities, reducing compliance, and reducing symptoms. Patient assessment must be done rigorously using different scales—mMRC, CAT, SaO2, cough questionnaires, spirometry, Dlco, BORG, 6MWT, and interdisciplinary consultations.

The COVID-19 pandemic has brought new challenges related to the need for social distancing to prevent the transmission of the infection so that long-encouraged online pulmonary rehabilitation is highly accessible, cheap, and has benefits, as demonstrated by numerous studies. In most cases, patients were delighted with this rehabilitation method and we can say that it remains a flexible option for those who cannot go to the hospital for various reasons.

The studies carried out over time comparing the two methods of rehabilitation—in the hospital and online at home showed favorable results in terms of increasing tolerance to effort, reducing symptoms, and increasing the level of physical activity, but a weak point it would be the fact that telerehabilitation has a limitation, namely the patients' ability to use the connecting devices, especially since we are talking about COPD, which is a pathology that appears in old age.

Conflict of interest

The authors declare no conflict of interest.

Author details

Paula Irina Barata[1,2*] and Maria Daniela Mot[1,2]

1 Western University "Vasile Goldiş" of Arad, Arad, Romania

2 Arad County Emergency Clinical Hospital, Arad, Romania

*Address all correspondence to: barata_paula@yahoo.com

References

[1] Halpin DMG, Celli BR, Criner GJ, Frith P, López Varela MV, Salvi S, et al. The GOLD Summit on Chronic Obstructive Pulmonary Disease in Low- and Middle-Income Countries. The International Journal of Tuberculosis and Lung Disease. 1 Nov 2019;**23**(11):1131-1141. DOI: 10.5588/ijtld.19.0397. PMID: 31718748

[2] Agusti A, Vogelmeier CF. GOLD 2024: A brief overview of key changes. J Bras Pneumol. 22 Dec 2023;**49**(6):e20230369. DOI: 10.36416/1806-3756/e20230369. PMID: 38126685; PMCID: PMC10760434

[3] McGinnis JM, Foege WH. Actual Causes of Death in the United States. Washington, DC: US Department of Health and Human Services; 2020

[4] Sharma BB, Singh V. Pulmonary rehabilitation: An overview. Lung India. Oct 2011;**28**(4):276-284. DOI: 10.4103/0970-2113.85690. PMID: 22084542; PMCID: PMC3213715

[5] NewsMed. Reabilitarea respiratorie-tehnici și indicații. 2024. Available from: https://newsmed.ro/reabilitarea-respiratorietehnici-si-indicatii

[6] Bourne S, DeVos R, North M, Chauhan A, Green B, Brown T, et al. Online versus face-to-face pulmonary rehabilitation for patients with chronic obstructive pulmonary disease: Randomised controlled trial. BMJ Open. 2017;**7**:e014580. DOI: 10.1136/bmjopen-2016-014580

[7] Raleigh M, Chang J, Virtual vs. In-person pulmonary rehabilitation for chronic lung disease. American Family Physician. 2022;**105**(2):135-136

[8] Tsutsui M, Gerayeli F, Sin DD. Pulmonary rehabilitation in a post-COVID-19 world: Telerehabilitation as a new standard in patients with COPD. International Journal of Chronic Obstructive Pulmonary Disease. 2021;**16**:379-391. DOI: 10.2147/COPD.S263031

[9] Seidman Z, McNamara R, Wootton S, Leung R, Spencer L, Dale M, et al. People attending pulmonary rehabilitation demonstrate a substantial engagement with technology and willingness to use telerehabilitation: A survey. Journal of Physiotherapy. 2017;**63**(3):175-181. DOI: 10.1016/j.jphys.2017.05.010. Epub 2017 Jun 23

[10] Spruit MA, Singh SJ, Garvey C, Zuwallack R, Nici L, Rochester C, et al. An official American Thoracic Society/European Respiratory Society statement: Key concepts and advances in pulmonary rehabilitation. American Journal of Respiratory and Critical Care Medicine. 2013;**188**(8):e13-e64. DOI: 10.1164/rccm.201309-1634ST. Erratum in: Am J Respir Crit Care Med. 2014 Jun 15;189(12):1570

[11] Okamoto J, Furukawa Y, Kobinata N, Yoshikawa H, Araki F, Yagyu A, et al. Combined effect of pulmonary rehabilitation and music therapy in patients with chronic obstructive pulmonary disease. Journal of Physical Therapy Science. 2021;**33**(10):779-783. DOI: 10.1589/jpts.33.779. Epub 2021 Oct 13

[12] Shi M, Yang L, Qumu S, Lei J, Huang K, He R, et al. Efficacy and safety of a music-therapy facilitated pulmonary telerehabilitation program in COPD patients: The COPDMELODY study protocol. Frontiers in Medicine (Lausanne). 8 Mar 2024;**11**:1361053. DOI: 10.3389/fmed.2024.1361053. PMID: 38523907; PMCID: PMC10957573

Chapter 6

Physical Activity: An Immunity Booster for Treating Respiratory Diseases

Qurat Ul Ain, Marian Gabriel, Irum Shahzad, Wajida Perveen, Ayesha Fiaz and Yasha Sajjad

Abstract

The interplay between physical activity and the immune system has garnered significant attention, especially in the context of respiratory diseases. Understanding this relationship is crucial, given the global burden of respiratory conditions such as COVID-19, influenza, and other upper respiratory tract infections (URTIs). This proposal aims to explore how physical activity can serve as an immunity booster and its potential in treating immunopathological conditions in respiratory diseases. The COVID-19 pandemic has further underscored the importance of maintaining physical activity to mitigate the adverse effects of prolonged inactivity on the immune system. Immobilization due to hospitalization and quarantine can downregulate immune responses, making individuals more susceptible to severe outcomes from respiratory infections. This research has the potential to inform public health recommendations and clinical practices aimed at leveraging physical activity as a non-pharmacological intervention to boost immunity and manage respiratory diseases. By establishing a clear connection between exercise and immune function, this study will contribute to the development of holistic treatment approaches for respiratory conditions, ultimately improving patient outcomes and reducing healthcare burdens.

Keywords: immunity, physical activity, respiratory illness, immobilization, holistic approach

1. Introduction

Physical activity has a powerful impact on the immune system, as it boosts preventive and recovery mechanisms in virtually all health scenarios. First, regular exercise increases immune surveillance by more T-cells and natural killer (NK) cells circulating, which makes it easier for the body to recognize these invading pathogens. This is the "J-curve" relationship, whereby moderate exercise strengthens immune function but intense prolonged activity impairs it through elevation of stress hormones such as cortisol.

In the longer term, habitual moderate-intensity exercise has been related to lower rates of upper respiratory tract infections (URTIs), proving its immunosuppressive effect. In the early or recovery stages of infections, easing back into a light activity may be beneficial to healing but needs careful moderation so as not to overwhelm an already stressed immune system. In immobile patients, either hospitalized or subjected to quarantine, early mobilization halts the immune deprivation induced by inactivity that leads to increased susceptibility to infections.

In patients with chronic respiratory diseases, exercise enhances pulmonary function and attenuates systemic inflammation by reducing plasma levels of pro-inflammatory mediators. The presence of both physical and psychological benefits highlights the need to incorporate physical activity into public health and clinical guidelines for immune and respiratory health [1].

2. Mechanisms of immune modulation through physical activity

Physical activity is defined as any movement that causes one to expend energy above basal levels, such as carrying out work, walking, or playing. When there is order and repetition with the aim of improving fitness level, it is termed physical exercise. Exercise, as a regime, may be classified as acute or chronic in nature. Acute exercises are quick and bring about physiological alterations like an enhanced heart rate or stirring immune cells into action. Conversely, chronic exercises bring about transformation due to changes in metabolism or lowered inflammation. Physiological responses are influenced by the intensity and volume of exercise undertaken with measurement of VO_{2max} offering crucial insights regarding aerobic fitness.

2.1 Physical activity vs. physical exercise

The word physical refers to any bodily movement produced by skeletal muscles and the energy expenses other than that of rest. It covers basic work activities such as house chores or construction work, means of transport like walking or cycling, as well as leisure activities such as dancing or playing sports. If physical activity is carried out in an organized and repetitive manner with the aim of enhancing one's fitness, it gets called physical exercise. Both physical activity and exercise are capable of eliciting acute or chronic effects, the latter being the eventual outcome of systematic physical training over time.

The magnitude and pattern of an individual muscle's contraction at any given moment influences the physiological response of any exercise performed as well as its effectiveness. One imperative factor determining the scope of muscular and cardiopulmonary systems during exercise is the often used term percentage of maximum oxygen uptake VO_2max. VO_2max is the term used to express the capability of the respiratory and cardiovascular system to supply oxygen to working muscles and muscles' capability to use it effectively. Viewed in non-exercising subjects, the untrained usually does about 15 times VO2 max where oxygen intake is 15 times in rest. For endurance athletes, this figure is 25 times higher [1].

2.2 Physiological attributes of physical activity

What happens in the body's homeostasis immediately following a single acute exercise session? According to research, rapid changes such as an increase in heart rate and a redistribution of immune cells typically occur. These acute responses are necessary to ensure the higher energy and oxygen requirements of a muscle that is contracting in some way. An energy "crunch" is created during muscular activity and leads to the production of reactive oxygen species (ROS), which is recognized as the stress signal. ROS at moderate level allows the body to adapt and reinforce antioxidant defenses; however, overproduction due to high intensity workouts contributes to severe oxidative stress which causes damage to cells and exacerbates inflammatory cytokines.

Chronic exercise puts pressure on certain muscles that over time creates biochemical adjustments such as improved metabolic efficiency and lowered levels of inflammation. Specialized and tailored exercises at a moderate frequency like aerobic exercises prevent an individual from stress by producing anti-inflammatory cytokines due to a decrease in oxidative stress, thus preventing inflammatory diseases even that of respiratory system. On the other hand, a lack of exercise does not seem to disturb the body condition greatly, and so, these improvements are not seen [2].

2.2.1 The dose: Response relationship between physical activity and health effects

Although it seems simple, the relationship between exercise and immune function is not straightforward; a comprehensive approach is required in creating an optimal exercise routine. Moderate intensity exercise improves immune compliance and decreases chronic inflammation; intensive or prolonged exercise, however, may exhibit effects opposite to that [1].

As for any medicine, there is also a dose–response relationship in physical activity and health outcomes. According to the J-curve hypothesis, there is clear relation between the volume of physical activity performed and benefits accrued from it: exercise has dose-dependent benefits, but usage of too much exercise serves to provide no benefits, and in many cases, even decreases in health outcomes. Moderate amounts of exercising will prevent and work against viral disease, and also allow for healthy metabolic control; however, intense exercising for extended periods can lead to reduced immune function, free radical imbalances, and other health hazards. As such, an ideal exercise program should be specifically tailored for the subject in question (**Figure 1**).

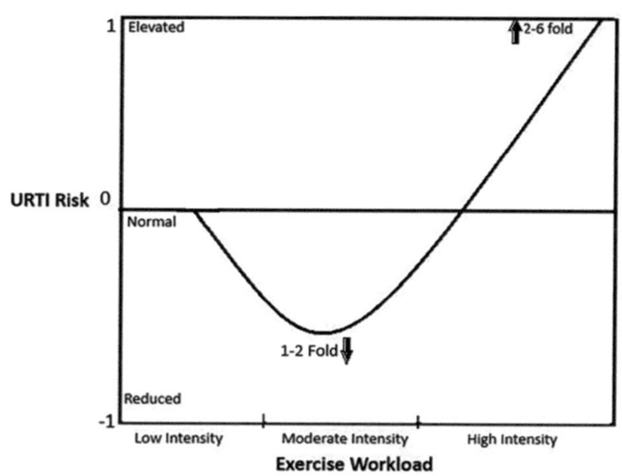

Figure 1.
J-curve relation between exercise intensity and immunity [3].

Regular exercise has strong benefits for the respiratory system, with moderate intensity exercise increasing both innate and adaptive immunity and subsequently decreasing the frequency and intensity of respiratory infections. However, athletes doing high volume training and training loads without adequate recovery may be more prone to respiratory infections during the "open-window" following heavy exercise. Apart from the immune system, regular moderate exercise has benefits of metabolic, cardiovascular, and neuro-endocrine health as well as decreases chronic inflammation and the risk of having cardiovascular diseases, type 2 diabetes, and neurodegenerative diseases. This dual effect of exercise on immune system and chronic inflammation suggests that exercise is one of the rare non-pharmacological modulations that can be utilized as an adjuvant to maintain health and manage chronic disorders [4].

2.3 The immune response to exercise

The body's response to infection or tissue damage is inflammation, as the body is designed to react to these stimuli. Its biological purpose is to assist in eliminating infections because of its active involvement in tissue reinstatement. Notwithstanding, when inflammation becomes distractingly chronic or disproportional, it is associated with a variety of diseases such as insulin resistance, diabetes, and cardiovascular diseases. The immune system is highly influenced by exercise and in particular the inflammation process.

If inflammation is in excess levels than what is needed in the body, moderate exercises can help stimulate a more balanced immune response; anti-inflammatory cytokine IL-10 can be produced, while pro-inflammatory cytokine TNF-α can be inhibited during moderate intensity exercises. When a person is exercising, different cells of the immune system, such as neutrophils and macrophages as well as natural killer cells (NK cells), are deployed into the blood stream, which increases immune's "eyes and ears" throughout circulation. This redistribution of immune cells to peripheral tissues enhances the effectiveness of the immune system, increasing its capacity to respond to new threats.

On the contrary, too much or too prolonged exercise can sequester native immune activity providing a temporary "window" of opportunity during which the acquired immune system can be intrinsically impaired. This span of time, around 1 to 2 h followed by exercise, has a lower level of presence of circulation containing lymphocytes that in turn could predispose the body to the danger of getting infections such as upper respiratory tract infections (URTIs) [5].

2.3.1 Open window theory

Physical exercise should not be regarded as a neutral activity since it has an impact on the immune system in a variable manner with respect to mode, intensity, and duration. Exercise requires energy and produces reactive oxygen species (ROS), which elicit immune responses that may be beneficial or harmful depending on the situation. Low to moderate intensity exercise has an anti-inflammatory effect that helps in reducing the chances of developing chronic diseases. Exercise lasting for longer periods or having increased intensity can also lead to an inflammatory response and decrease the immune response. The "open-window" theory postulates that with intense training, there is an immune suppression that lasts for the short term and makes the host more prone to some infections such as upper

DOI: http://dx.doi.org/10.5772/intechopen.1008423

respiratory tract infections (URTIs). For the first 1 to 2 h after exercise, there is assumed to be a temporal alteration that decreases the immune response that increases the risk of infections. This confusion is fueled by the fact that some believe this immune-suppression may be an immune response, as rest is geographically restrained immune cells to the sites of higher infection risks like the lungs and the gastrointestinal tract [6].

2.3.2 Innate and adaptive immune responses

The innate immune system, fundamental to the body's first line of defense against infection, has been shown to be involved in the immune response to exercise.

Aerobic exercise correlates with an increase in functional NK cells, neutrophils, and macrophages, which are components of innate immunity; moderate intensity exercise recruits these cells to new locations in the body for better infection prevention. However, after vigorous exercise, immune cells are often circulated out of the blood stream, and this phenomenon is consistent with the "open window" hypothesis. This relocalization decreases the absolute numbers of immune cells in the blood and, in the short term, creates the risk of infections including upper respiratory tract infections (URTIs). Postexercise neutrophils and macrophages are crucial for infection clearance but have shown to decrease in circulation cells but migrate to infected tissues, which suggest that there is a focal immune system protective response that might compensate for the loss in circulation.

The adaptive immune response mediated by lymphocytes as well as the production of antibodies is also mediated by exercise. Intense physical exercise seems to be associated with a dramatic increase in T- and B-lymphocytes populations, which implies some kind of stimulus on the immune system. This is then succeeded by a transient drop in peripheral blood lymphocyte numbers, a phenomenon known as lymphopenia. Instead of indicating immune system suppression, this event triggers gene expression in T-cells to those locations rather than inhibition of peripheral T-cells which induces lymphopenia.

Cytokines are also influenced by the level of exertion given. Such as in high-intensity exercise activity, pro-inflammatory cytokines like interferon gamma (IFN-γ) and tumor necrosis factor alpha (TNF-α) are secreted that stimulate the pathway of immune response. However, regular and moderate exercise induces the secretion of anti-inflammatory cytokines including interleukin-10 (IL-10) to help control the immune system and reduce chronic inflammation. The ROS is stated as another word for oxidative stress and is toxic and damaging to living organisms and self-cells. However, the moderate level of ROS produced through moderate exercise aids antioxidant level and immune balance in the body. Yet abuse of exertion in the form of high-intensity or long periods of exercise leads to excessive production of ROS that are harmful and lead to chronic inflammation and oxidative stress. The aerobic fitness enhances the capacity to replenish tissues, that is, muscle and the pre-exercise environment switches from anti to pro-inflammatory helping further strengthen recovery of the immune system. All these processes happen in response to physical activity with presence of both types of mediators in the end.

These kinds of inflammatory processes in the body are of utmost importance especially during- post tissue damage when microbes or structures associated with pathogens are recognized and destroy the microbial community. In addition, damage-associated molecular patterns (DAMPs) released by injured or dying cells prompt further immune activation that assists in tissue repair and recovery [7].

3. Effect of physical activity on acute RTI

Acute respiratory infections (ARIs) are perhaps among the most notable etiological health problems, which contribute to both morbidity and mortality throughout the world. Routine health check-ups and days spent on sick leave are often due to ARIs that include "common cold" and influenza whereas; more serious sections like pneumonia may even require a person to go to hospital or may cause death in certain at-risk groups. The scope for the development of newer preventative measures such as physical exercise has also come out quite strongly in light of the COVID-19 pandemic, which has been exceptional in terms of the damage caused by respiratory diseases to society.

Many studies have shown that the rate of ARIs has been inversely associated with the level of physical activity of the people, that is, the more physically active individuals, the lower the frequency of ARIs. A study suggests that adults who are physically active with moderate-to-vigorous intensity are able to decrease the frequency and intensity of cold-related symptoms by 46% during the study period. Other studies of similar nature highlight that the risk of ARIs, particularly pneumonia, was reported to be 31% lower among the physically active suggesting that exercise will help strengthen immune system applicability towards fighting off viral and bacterial infections. As many studies have shown the effect, the causative factors that have also been explored include the diseased population of coronary heart disease and diabetic population that have reported reduced hospital visits when they maintain suggested levels of physical health.

3.1 COVID-19

Another global health emergency: Today's COVID-19 pandemic and many other conditions such as influenza and pneumonia can be classified and ranked as top most death-causing diseases, and all of them can be said to have an inverse relation with physical activity. In a large cohort study, it was found that patients that followed both aerobic and muscle-strengthening workouts were at a 54% lower risk of dying from these infections compared to those that remained inactive. This reduction was higher than what is noted for chronic illness and cardiovascular diseases, which indicates the need for exercise in those with deteriorating conditions.

This had some other helpful side effects, which are also sustainable (as in sustainably positive). A two-year large cohort retrospective study conducted in the United Kingdom found on its outcomes that patients who met the MVPA guidelines were associated with significantly lower risks of hospitalization due to severe COVID-19 or ICU admission. One analysis determined that adverse health results of COVID-19 were increased by 149% in inactive individuals compared to physical activity recommendation adherence. It should, however, be noted that not all types of exercises included in the investigation prevented an SARS-CoV-2 infection. Some others suggested moderate doses of workouts lead to a slight positive effect reducing COVID-19 infection but restrained spreading. The results are also consistent with the finding that physical activity may help control disease severity but not prevent initiation.

While the vast majority of high-quality evidence has supported physical activity to reduce risk for ARIs, implementations in the public health policies have not kept pace. The CDC has very recently said that they knew there were more factors, but just added inactivity to the list of high risk behaviors for severe COVID-19 adverse outcomes. Other commentaries are echoing the sentiment for ARI prevention as a part of public health guidelines, further bolstering the "Exercise is Medicine" initiative that extols physical activity as an important armament in combating not just chronic disease but also infectious illness [8].

4. Effect of physical activity on chronic RTI

Engaging in physical activity and structured exercise is recognized as a powerful, non-pharmacological measure of prevention and management of a number of chronic diseases. A significant number of studies serve as evidence of the fact that higher levels of your physical activity are associated with better health, particularly due to musculoskeletal, cardiopulmonary, metabolic, sleep, cognitive, and pain management system improvements. In addition, exercise is an important factor to be considered in the management of disease with acute or chronic immune activation as it alters immune response.

4.1 Chronic obstructive pulmonary disease

Chronic obstructive pulmonary disease (COPD) is a long-term lung condition that causes airflow to progressively decrease accompanied by persistent cough and dyspnea limiting physical capacity and quality of life. Inevitably, this entails greater risk of cardiovascular disease (CVD), which is an important contributor to the increased mortality among COPD. Many patients with COPD experience physical inactivity, which is a consequence of breathing problems, tiredness, and muscle function impairment. This inactivity, in turn, only causes more health problems, perpetuating a cycle of worsening symptoms and cardiovascular strain that can ultimately increase mortality. This vicious cycle can be interrupted with regular physical activity, as improvements in cardiovascular health, lung capacity, and physical integrity are all important factors associated with COPD.

Even low to moderate volumes of habitual exercise can substantially reduce all-cause mortality in this group. Physical activity improves heart rate, blood pressure, and vascular function that are often impaired in patients with COPD, and thereby, exercise reduces cardiovascular load. Consequently, it causes a decrease in the risk of heart disease (a common comorbidity and a leading cause of death in COPD, which is achieved by decreasing cardiovascular stress. Also, regular exercise helps control comorbidities (hypertension and diabetes), which in turn reduces mortality.

People who are physically active (PA) regularly live longer than those who sensibly stay away from PA. Physical activity enhances the working capacity of both the lungs and muscles, which can help COPD patients better, carry out daily tasks, and live independently [9].

4.2 Asthma

Asthma, as a chronic pulmonary disease with acute bouts of airway inflammation and constriction, results in symptoms such as wheezing, breathlessness, and coughing. Standard protocol for treating asthma typically emphasizes pharmacological interventions like inhaled corticosteroids and bronchodilators to control symptoms and prevent flare-ups. However, incorporating physical exercise into asthma management can surely enhance patient outcomes by taking into account both the physical and psychological dimensions of the disease.

Regular moderate-intensity physical exercise offers multiple reimbursements for individuals with asthma. It can improve cardiopulmonary fitness, lessen systemic inflammation, and improve the whole quality of life. While asthma patients may choose not to exercise because primary asthma symptoms get triggered or EIB may occur, but still, exercise helps in the long-term control of asthma. Physical exercise enhances respiratory muscle strength and function and also decreases inflammation within the airways and, correspondingly, rate of exacerbations. Also, physical exercise plays a role in weight loss since obesity produces poor asthma outcomes and contributes to disease control complications. Physical exercise shows little, if any, positive impact on lung functions or eradicating asthma, but the exercise boosts the cardiovascular and muscular endurance, which makes patients have better control in handling flares. Moreover, physical activity has positive impacts on the mental health of patients, including decreased levels of anxiety and depression that are often elevated in asthmatics. Mental health in turn reduces stress and symptom precipitation of asthma; hence, patients get a stronger feeling of managing their illness. In order to obtain the most favorable outcome from physical activity, it is suggested to use exercise programs depending on a patient's level of asthma control and physical activity. Recommendations like warm-up, stretching, using short-acting bronchodilators, and a gradual buildup to exercise can prevent EIB. This applies equally to the educational functions of interventions as to the influence of patients' fear regarding exercise; the approach helps maintain a proper level of activity without leading to overstress [10].

5. Exercise in hospitalized and quarantined patients

Many patients discharged from a hospital setting can appropriately understand the need for care for the underlying condition that forced hospitalization. However, some may become dependent on care due to the most often unrecognized out-turn in even well managed underlying diseases, which is functional decline. This is commonly referred to as hospital associated functional decline (HAFD) when there is a drop of the ability to perform activities of daily living (ADLs) such as eating or dressing oneself. About 30% of all older adults admitted to a hospital are reported to suffer from this deficiency which higher the chances of subsequent disability, living in institutions, or even death. Hospitalization also poses a threat to cognition and exposes one to an increased risk of dementia and cognitive decline, calling for measures that must be taken to prevent adverse consequences.

One logistics weakness that explains the risk factors of such illness includes low amounts of physical activities while in the hospital. Although many of the admitted patients are physically able to ambulate, they do remain largely bedridden throughout the time there. About 75% of older outpatients in hospitals are shown to not walk at all in the duration of stay. As a result, rapid muscle wasting, loss of motion, as well as recurrent respiratory infections and normalization of conditions increase. This immobility, in addition to the psychosocial stress associated with being in hospital, would have devastating effects and delays recovery and chances of being readmitted to the hospital or even death [11].

In light of these concerns, exercise interventions are increasingly becoming the cornerstone of avoiding further deterioration in the physical abilities of hospitalized patients. Suitable mobile rehabilitation programs — that is, preventative rehabilitation directed at medically stable patients — promote mobility, enable activities of daily living, and reduce institutionalization rates. Meta-analytic studies are conclusive that physical activity performed after discharging a patient from a hospital leads to better health outcomes and lowers mortality risks. More evidence is coming forth that starting to exercise programs in the hospital setting may also mitigate a patient's functional decline, improve his physical capacity, and increase his level of independence at the time of discharge [12].

Nevertheless, the provision of exercise programs in the hospital does come with certain issues. Most hospitalized patients will have numerous chronic diseases that makes it difficult to come up with appropriate exercise programs. Furthermore, the acute healthcare providers' attention should be mainly placed at dealing with what we will call the primary medical condition as well as lack of emphasis on mobility and rehabilitation during the hospitalization period. There is a workaround to this; hospitals need to design easy, uncomplicated exercises that would not strain or put the patients at risk. Working together with the physicians, physiotherapist, and the rehabilitation specialists alike is very important for the effectiveness of these interventions [11].

6. Correlation between psychological and immunological aspects of exercise

Physical activity, chiefly in the form of prolonged exercise such as treadmill walking or cycling, has been revealed to significantly adjust symptoms of depression and anxiety in individuals suffering from chronic obstructive pulmonary disease (COPD). This improvement is for the most part attributable to the stabilization of the hypothalamic–pituitary–adrenal (HPA) axis, which in turn leads to a reduction in cortisol levels and settles systemic inflammation, both of which are common contributors to the experience of depression in chronic conditions. Furthermore, regular physical activity not only diminishes negative emotional states by providing mental distractions; however, it also enhances muscle strength and functional capacity, thereby improving the overall quality of life. The reduction in cortisol production, a hormone majorly associated with stress, has shown to play a crucial role in this process, as it supports healthier muscle metabolism and limits muscle loss. Interestingly, although training benefits are observable across various age groups, the response to exercise can differ based on factors such as gender, age, and training intensity. This suggests a necessity for tailored exercise regimens to maximize benefits.

These findings underscored the potential of physical exercise, not merely for physical health but also as a therapeutic modality for managing depression and anxiety in patients with chronic diseases. However, this dual benefit is often overlooked, primarily because many individuals fail to recognize the profound psychological advantages that physical activity can yield. Although exercise is frequently associated with improved physical well-being, its role in enhancing mental health is equally significant. This comprehensive understanding is crucial for healthcare providers aiming to adopt a holistic approach to patient treatment [13].

7. Guidelines for physical activity in respiratory health promotion and immunity

Some researchers estimate that there are about 117 million Americans that include one or more preventable chronic diseases. Physical activity has a beneficial impact on seven out of the 10 most widespread chronic diseases according to the World Health Organization. Physical activity recommendations related to aerobic health-enhancing activity are not met by nearly 80 percent of the adults, while only about half of the adults meet the key guidelines for aerobic physical activity. The lack of physical activity in the population is related to approximately 117 billion dollars in healthcare expenditures annually and about a 10 percent decline in average lifespan of humans [14].

Attempting to exercise vigorously is inherently risky and may escalate the prevalence of adverse cardiovascular as well as pulmonary events, primarily among individuals who already are on the verge of associated risk factors. The importance of such a risk highlights the need for individually tailored exercise protocols taking into account their medical condition, fitness level, and goals. Following the minimum recommended levels of physical activity is beneficial to health; however, more active individuals are likely to also gain further health and fitness improvements. But at the same time, it is important to find balance so that one is not harmed by being too vigorous [1].

7.1 Physical activity guidelines for Americans

The Physical Activity Guidelines for Americans (2024) emphasize that to achieve health benefits from exercise, there has to be progression, overload, and specificity: these are some of the principles of training. Progression measures the ability to gradually advance the intensity or duration of a particular exercise. Overload considers burdening the body in more amounts than is customary in order to promote the adaptation within its cells and tissues. Specificity is understood in terms of the compliance of the exercises done with the end goal, such as improved aerobic capacity, muscle strength, and even joint flexibility. The absence of at least one of these can greatly reduce the health benefits that come from exercising.

There is scientific evidence that light to moderate physical activity, especially walking and cycling lasting for 5 to 15 min for 2 to 3 times a week, is associated with low risks of serious musculoskeletal injuries and other known cardiovascular events. In view of the wide range of options regarding an activity level, individuals should consider their age, current fitness status, and previous experience in physical activities when progressing in plans of activities [14].

7.2 WHO guidelines for COVID-19 patients

Patients diagnosed with moderate to severe COVID-19 infections require admission to the hospital, oxygen therapy, and ICU management, especially in the presence of sepsis, acute respiratory distress syndrome (ARDS), or multi-organ failure. Patients with invasive mechanical ventilation are faced with muscle weakness, impaired physical functioning, and alteration in breathing pattern as a result of sedation and prolonged bed rest, and various other challenges. Negative consequences like post ICU syndrome may result in low exercise tolerance, incapability in performing activities of daily living and poor quality of life, as well as their susceptibility for other respiratory infections for months or years following their discharge from the hospital (**Table 1**) [15].

7.3 Global initiative for asthma (GINA) guidelines

In the general population, including asthmatics, regular moderate-level physical exercise confers important health benefits including decreased cardiovascular risk

COVID-19 patients undergo rehabilitation interventions on three levels: acute, subacute, and long-term recovery.		
Phase	**Interventions**	**Site of care**
Acute	• Assistance in respiratory management (oxygenation, chest clearance, and ventilation weaning) • Maintain proper nutrition • Prevent complications (aspiration pneumonia)	ICU, CCU, HDU
Sub-Acute	• Early mobilization • Breathing exercises • Introduce independence for ADLs • Provide psychosocial support	Hospital wards, step-down facilities
Chronic	• Practice graded exercise • Energy conservation techniques • Respiratory rehab	Outpatient department, rehab centers, home services

Table 1.
WHO guidelines for COVID-19 Rehabilitation [15].

and improved quality of life. When it comes to chronic respiratory illness, exercise and physical activity have no particular effect on lung function or asthma symptoms, but increased cardiopulmonary fitness may be associated with a decreased likelihood of misdiagnosed exercise-induced dyspnea not attributable to airflow limitation as in asthma. According to GINA –2019, in nonobese individuals with asthma found improvements in levels of asthma symptom control after a combined high-protein, low-glycemic index diet, and high-intensity interval training, but no effect on lung function. Swimming training is well tolerated and improves lung function and cardiopulmonary fitness in young asthma populations; although, contact with chlorine in indoor pools is of concern.

In many patients, especially those with EIB, exercise is a common evocative factor for their asthma symptoms, but when exercise-induced breakthrough symptoms do arise, they are often well-controlled with a warm-up before exercising, or SABA or low-dose inhaled corticosteroid-formoterol taken in advance of and/or during physical activity. At this stage of the research, there is insufficient evidence to determine whether particular forms of physical activity are more advantageous than others. Nevertheless, physical activity does not offer targeted benefits in terms of lung function or asthma symptoms with the sole exception being swimming in children with asthma [16].

8. Conclusion

Besides maintaining general health, exercise is an immunity booster most significant for dealing with acute as well as chronic pulmonary infections. The immune response in general is enhanced when one takes moderate exercise; this conveys an increased traffic of other immune competent cells including the versatile T-cells and natural killer cells whose function is to patrol the body in search of pathogens.

Physical activity also helps to decrease the degrees of inflammatory markers including IL-6/TNF-α to bring about a highly efficient immune setting. In the same manner, it enhances lung capacity and respiratory muscle strength that are so vital to patients with, or susceptible to respiratory illness. In this perspective, stress and anxiety are lowered by exercise, and cortisol, a stress hormone that negatively affects the immune system, is also controlled. Collectively, these advantages make physical activity an efficient approach for enhancing immunity and shielding against respiratory ailments, thus enhancing both the short-term and chronic well-being.

Author details

Qurat Ul Ain[1]*, Marian Gabriel[1], Irum Shahzad[1], Wajida Perveen[3], Ayesha Fiaz[4] and Yasha Sajjad[2]

1 Riphah International University, Lahore, Pakistan

2 DPT School of Allied Health Sciences, Combined Military Hospital, Lahore Medical College and Institute of Dentistry (NUMS), Lahore, Pakistan

3 Department of Physical Therapy, CMH Lahore Medical College and Institute of Dentistry (NUMS), Lahore, Pakistan

4 DHQ hospital Sheikhupura, Pakistan

*Address all correspondence to: qurat.ain@riphah.edu.pk

References

[1] da Luz SD, Latini A. Exercise-induced immune system response: Anti-inflammatory status on peripheral and central organs. Biochimicaet Biophysica Acta (BBA)-Molecular Basis of Disease. 2020;**1866**(10):165823. DOI: 10.1016/j.bbadis.2020.165823

[2] Filgueira TO, Castoldi A, Santos LER, de Amorim GJ, de Sousa Fernandes MS, Anastácio WDLDN, et al. The relevance of a physical active lifestyle and physical fitness on immune defense: Mitigating disease burden, with focus on COVID-19 consequences. Frontiers in Immunology. 2021;**12**:587146. DOI: 10.3389/fimmu.2021.587146

[3] Nieman DC, Wentz LM. The compelling link between physical activity and the body's defense system. Journal of Sport and Health Science. 2019;**8**(3):201-217. DOI: 10.1016/j.jshs.2018.09.009

[4] Sabzevari RR. The impact of different training intensities on athletes' immune system function and the management of upper respiratory traction infections: A narrative review. Sport Sciences for Health. 2024;**20**(2):415-426. DOI: 10.1007/s11332-023-01110-7

[5] Campbell JP, Turner JE. Debunking the myth of exercise-induced immune suppression: Redefining the impact of exercise on immunological health across the lifespan. Frontiers in Immunology. 2018;**9**:648. DOI: 10.3389/fimmu.2018.00648

[6] Ranasinghe C, Ozemek C, Arena R. Exercise and well-being during COVID 19–time to boost your immunity. Expert Review of Anti-Infective Therapy. 2020;**18**(12):1195-1200. DOI: 10.1080/14787210.2020.1794818

[7] Von AH, Morano AE, Dorneles GP, Peres A, Lira FS. The role of glucose homeostasis on immune function in response to exercise: The impact of low or higher energetic conditions. Journal of Cellular Physiology. 2020;**235**(4):3169-3188. DOI: 10.1002/jcp.29228

[8] Nieman DC, Sakaguchi CA. Physical activity lowers the risk for acute respiratory infections: Time for recognition. Journal of Sport and Health Science. 2022;**11**(6):648-655. DOI: 10.1016/j.jshs.2022.08.002

[9] Shu C-C, Lee J-H, Tsai M-K, Su T-C, Wen CP. The ability of physical activity in reducing mortality risks and cardiovascular loading and in extending life expectancy in patients with COPD. Scientific Reports. 2021;**11**(1):21674. DOI: 10.1038/s41598-021-00728-2

[10] Panagiotou M, Koulouris NG, Rovina N. Physical activity: A missing link in asthma care. Journal of Clinical Medicine. 2020;**9**(3):706. DOI: 10.3390/jcm9030706

[11] Valenzuela PL, Morales JS, Castillo-García A, Mayordomo-Cava J, García-Hermoso A, Izquierdo M, et al. Effects of exercise interventions on the functional status of acutely hospitalised older adults: A systematic review and meta-analysis. Ageing Research Reviews. 2020;**61**:101076. DOI: 10.1016/j.arr.2020.101076

[12] Schujmann DS, Gomes TT, Lunardi AC, Lamano MZ, Fragoso A, Pimentel M, et al. Impact of a progressive mobility program on the functional status, respiratory, and muscular systems of ICU patients: A randomized and controlled trial. Critical Care Medicine. 2020;**48**(4):491-497. DOI: 10.1097/CCM.0000000000004181

[13] Ismail A. Stress axis response to aerobic exercise in chronic obstructive pulmonary disease patients. Advances in Rehabilitation. 2022;**36**(4):24-32. DOI: 10.5114/areh.2022.123180

[14] Olson RD, Vaux-Bjerke A, Quam JB, Piercy KL, Troiano RP, George SM, et al. Physical activity guidelines for Americans. Nadar! Swimming Magazine. 2023;**3**(166):9-10. Available from: https://www.revistanadar.com.br/index.php/Swimming-Magazine/article/view/48 [Accessed: November 10, 2024]

[15] Pan American Health Organization. Rehabilitation Considerations During the COVID-19 Outbreak [Internet]. 2020. Available from: https://iris.paho.org/handle/10665.2/52035 [Accessed: November 10, 2024]

[16] GINA Main Report. Global Strategy for Asthma Management and Prevention [Internet]. 2019. Available from: https://ginasthma.org/wp-content/uploads/2023/04/GINA-Main-Report-2019-WMSA.pdf [Accessed: November 10, 2024]

Chapter 7

Serum Amyloid A and Lipid Metabolism in Idiopathic Pulmonary Fibrosis: A New Target for Antifibrotic Therapy?

Lucia Vietri

Abstract

Lipid metabolism has been demonstrated to be altered in different interstitial lung diseases (ILDs), including idiopathic pulmonary fibrosis (IPF); it can influence the pathogenesis of fibrotic lung disorders. Serum Amyloid A (SAA) is an acute-phase protein mainly produced by the liver in response to proinflammatory cytokines. Several studies I conducted on Serum Amyloid A (SAA) support the hypothesis that this protein could be considered a potential specific biomarker for Idiopathic Pulmonary Fibrosis (IPF), capable of predicting the clinical course and prognosis of patients. SAA may help discriminate between a pulmonary interstitial disease with an inflammatory substrate and progressive pulmonary fibrosis. The follow-up of serum SAA levels over time could help us monitor the clinical and functional progression of IPF patients, as well as their risk of acute exacerbation, aiming to guide these patients toward antifibrotic therapies and lung transplantation within the appropriate time window. Additionally, my research on Serum Amyloid A reinforces the hypothesis of the role of lipid metabolism in the fibrogenic process. SAA plays a crucial role in regulating lipid metabolism and the production of matrix metalloproteinases (MMPs) in IPF, which are involved in extracellular matrix remodeling. SAA could be considered a potential therapeutic target for IPF, including through apolipoproteins.

Keywords: IPF, lipid metabolism, HDL cholesterol, SAA, biomarker

1. Introduction

1.1 Definition of serum amyloid A (SAA)

In response to injury or trauma, the liver is capable of releasing serum amyloid A protein, stimulated by acute-phase cytokines. SAA shares antigenicity with amyloid A, the major constituent of the fibrillar component in amyloidosis [1, 2]. SAA has been measured in serum and bronchoalveolar lavage (BAL) in various respiratory diseases (chronic inflammatory, neoplastic, and infectious). The potential clinical value of SAA as a biomarker for different lung diseases is the main topic of this chapter.

1.2 Protein structure and metabolism of SAA

Four genes on chromosome 11 have been identified in the human genome responsible for the synthesis of SAA1, SAA2, SAA3, and SAA4 [3]. The two acute-phase protein isoforms of SAA are encoded by the SAA1 and SAA2 genes; the tertiary structure of SAA is unknown, although the crucial role of the 10 amino-terminal residues in the formation of amyloid fibrils that bind high-density lipoprotein (HDL) is well established [3–6]. Serum amyloid A is synthesized also by macrophages, endothelial cells, smooth muscle cells, adipocytes, atherosclerotic lesions, and tumor cells [4, 7]. Upon release of A-SAA from cells, the protein binds HDL cholesterol and enters the bloodstream; this complex SAA-HDL is rapidly sequestered by phagocytes and broken down by lysosomal proteinases (serine proteases, elastase, collagenase, and cathepsins) [8–10].

1.3 Role of SAA in inflammation and in connective tissue diseases with lung involvement

In inflammatory diseases, plasma concentrations of SAA have been shown to be thousands of times higher than the baseline value. Serum SAA levels rise three to six hours after an inflammatory stimulus, and it normalizes after approximately three days. During acute inflammation, the main proteins released in response to cytokine stimulation (TNF-α, IL-1, and IL-6) are SAA and C-reactive protein (CRP) [11]. The serum concentration of SAA can reach thousands of mg/L, depending on the severity of the inflammatory process. Furthermore, SAA is considered more reliable than CRP, as its levels normalize after those of CRP, allowing differentiation between infectious, neoplastic, or autoimmune processes [2]. In patients with systemic sclerosis (SSc), some studies have shown that serum SAA concentration correlates with pulmonary involvement, which is associated with an unfavorable prognosis: they were inversely correlated with diffusing capacity of the lung for carbon monoxide (DLCO) rates, suggesting that SAA may be a biomarker of interstitial lung involvement in SSc patients [12]. The gene expression of SAA in patients with rheumatoid arthritis (RA) has been related to the transcription of extracellular matrix metalloproteinases. Increased concentrations of SAA have been found in synovial tissue in patients with rheumatoid arthritis [13–17].

1.4 SAA as a biomarker of acute exacerbation of chronic obstructive pulmonary diseases

Chronic obstructive pulmonary disease (COPD) is a disease characterized by persistent airflow limitation associated with chronic inflammation of the airways caused by agents, such as cigarette smoke, toxic gases, or even genetic predisposition. COPD presents with varying levels of severity depending on the degree of functional obstruction and clinical impairment of the patient. Acute exacerbation phases may occur, characterized by increased cough, sputum production/color, worsening dyspnea, requiring an increase in systemic and inhaled steroid therapy, and, in some cases, the use of antibiotic therapy and oxygen therapy. In severe cases, hospitalization is necessary. SAA and CRP levels rise during acute exacerbations of COPD due to the release of cytokines from the inflammatory cascade (IL-6, IL-1β, and TNF-α). SAA has also been proposed as a marker for acute exacerbation of COPD [18–20].

1.5 SAA in OSAS

A patient with obstructive sleep apnea syndrome (OSAS) exhibits significant snoring, a frequency of nocturnal apneas/hypopneas of varying severity, leading to poor sleep quality, daytime sleepiness, difficulty concentrating, and cardiovascular complications (secondary to the hypoxic condition). It is precisely the hypoxic state that induces an inflammatory response with the release of inflammatory mediators, including SAA and CRP. It has been shown that serum concentrations of SAA are higher in patients with severe OSAS than in those with mild or moderate OSAS. After 3 months of continuous positive airway pressure (CPAP), SAA levels decreased significantly in patients, with OSAS, along with parameters of cardiovascular risk and inflammation [21–23].

1.6 SAA in sarcoidosis

SAA induces the production of some cytokines and regulates T-helper1 (Th-1) lymphocytes in the immune response through interaction with the toll-like receptor 2 (TLR-2). Increased serum levels of SAA have been reported in patients with active sarcoidosis [24]. Unlike angiotensin-converting enzyme (ACE), the production of SAA is not inhibited by immunosuppressive drugs and its use has been recommended during the follow-up of patients with sarcoidosis [25]. SAA is expressed by macrophages and giant cells of sarcoid granulomas; it is found within granulomas and is expressed by CD68+ macrophages and giant cells [26]. Because it is an innate regulator of granulomatous inflammation that occurs in sarcoidosis through TLR-2, it offers new therapeutic targets.

SAA is involved in the formation of the sarcoid granuloma (likely following an initial mycobacterial infection). Furthermore, once released into circulation, SAA is able to bind to the isoform 3 of HDL, replacing apolipoprotein A1. The formation of this SAA-HDL3 complex results in reduced HDL concentrations in active sarcoidosis, making it a potential marker of disease activity [24, 27–29].

1.7 SAA in bronchial asthma

Bronchial asthma is a heterogeneous disease characterized by chronic airway inflammation with reversible bronchial obstruction (either spontaneously or following inhaled therapy). In allergic asthma, elevated serum levels of SAA have been recorded, likely in response to the cytokine cascade (IL-1β, IL-6, and IL-23) of the Th17 response [30–33].

1.8 SAA in lung cancer

SAA is known as an acute-phase protein involved in carcinogenesis. Elevated CRP levels have been reported to have prognostic significance in lung cancer patients, and a single study demonstrated increased CRP-SAA levels in lung cancer patients [34]. Lung cancer cells have higher expression of SAA1-SAA2 than normal lung cells, in turn, the neoplastic cells release IL-6, which induces the hepatic release of SAA. SAA, in turn, increases the expression of MMP-9, which is involved in the metastasis process. Higher concentrations of SAA are associated with lung cancer and the protein can therefore be suggested as a therapeutic target to prevent lung cancer metastasis [35–40].

1.9 SAA and SARS-COV-2

SAA serum levels were analyzed in some studies on patients affected by acute COVID-19.

SARS-COV-2 infection increases the SAA amyloid formation; overexpression of SAA does not always lead to systemic amyloidosis. SARS-COV-2 proteins can increase the risk of SAA fibril formation by these mechanisms:

- binding to the viral surface protein SK-9, it induces structural instability (from hexamer to monomer);
- an enzymatic cleavage transform monomers in smaller fragments that are found in SAA fibrils.

The presence of the viral protein SK-9 increases the risk of amyloid fibrils formations and deposition in the blood vessels, causing inflammation and thrombosis. It leads to the multisystem inflammatory syndrome observed in patients with severe COVID-19 with cardiovascular, gastrointestinal, dermatologic, and neurological symptoms [41]. Patients with severe COVID-19 have diffuse alveolar damage, which produces multiple inflammatory factors (IL-1, IL-6) that can rapidly induce a 1000-fold increase in SAA serum levels (198,32 mg/l). This biomarker was significantly higher in patients with critical COVID-19 [42, 43].

After his release, SAA binds HDL cholesterol and this complex induces the neutrophil activation aggravating the degree of inflammation and leading to the worsening of the patient.

2. Serological analysis project of SAA in IPF

To date, very few data are available in the literature regarding SAA and its potential role in Idiopathic Pulmonary Fibrosis (IPF), which is known to be the worst form of fibrosing interstitial lung disease, as it is associated with a poor prognosis and a survival rate of less than 5 years. IPF presents radiologically with a *Usual Interstitial Pneumonia* (UIP) pattern of pulmonary fibrosis; some patients have a stable form, also favored by the use of new antifibrotic drugs, while other patients have rapidly progressive variants with phases of acute acceleration and very rapid clinical progression. To date, we do not have a marker of severity and prognosis capable of establishing the evolution early and being able to send patients early to lung transplantation. The prognosis of IPF patients has significantly improved with the introduction of antifibrotic therapies (Pirfenidone and Nintedanib), which are able to slow disease progression as much as possible, thereby increasing life expectancy. It would therefore be valuable to identify new biomarkers that enable early diagnosis of IPF and allow monitoring of patients to identify those with an unstable, rapidly progressive phenotype.

2.1 First study of SAA in IPF

In 2019, together with my research group from the University of Siena, we enrolled 21 patients with IPF (14 male, mean age 64.8 ± 8 years) who were being followed up at the University of Siena, Respiratory Department. The diagnosis of IPF in the enrolled patients was made after discussion within the multidisciplinary team (pulmonologist, radiologist, rheumatologist, pathologist, bronchoscopist), in accordance with ATS/ERS/JRS/ALAT guidelines [44]. Clinical, functional, and immunological data were collected from all patients. Laboratory parameters included complete blood count with leukocyte differential, lipid profile, coagulation profile, lymphocyte typing on peripheral venous blood, serum protein electrophoresis, and iron status. The enrolled patients underwent functional monitoring of forced expiratory volume in 1 s (FEV1), forced vital capacity (FVC), total lung capacity (TLC), diffusing capacity of the lung for carbon monoxide (DLCO, absolute values expressed in milliliters and as percentage of predicted) every 6 months. Patients with OSAS, those on statin therapy, and those with significant cardiovascular diseases were excluded (as such conditions could have falsified the serum levels of SAA). The serum concentration of SAA was also analyzed in a control group of 11 healthy volunteers (3 male; mean age 55 ± 11.3 years), who were not taking any medications. All patients enrolled in the study provided informed consent to participate, in accordance with the guidelines established by the ethics committee of the University of Siena. SAA was analyzed in the laboratory using the ELISA (enzyme-linked immunosorbent assay) technique. All data are expressed as the mean ± standard deviation and the statistical analysis was performed with nonparametric tests. For statistical significance we used the Mann-Whitney U test; correlations between variables were analyzed through the Spearman correlation index (r) and survival was estimated using Kaplan-Meier curves. A p-value 0.05 was considered statistically significant.

The demographic characteristics of the enrolled population are detailed in **Table 1**.

The patients with IPF were older, with a significant predominance of men with a moderate restrictive deficit. Compared to the healthy control group, IPF patients exhibited significantly higher serum levels of SAA ($p = 0.003$) (**Figure 1**).

The data also revealed that SAA levels are not influenced by sex and a cut-off with a high AUC [area under the receiver operating characteristic (ROC) curve], 90.91% specificity for a cut-off value of 6067 ng/ml.

There was a negative correlation between SAA and HDL ($r = -6224$, $p = 0.0307$) and a significant inverse correlation between SAA and FVC percentage ($r = -0.5229$, $p = 0.0150$; **Figure 2**).

	IPF	HC	p-value
n	21	11	
Male (%)	14(66)	3(27)	0.03
Age (years)	64.8 ± 8.1	55 ± 11.3	0.01
Former smoker	16(76)	7(63)	0.45
Never smoker	5(24)	4(37)	0.45
FVC % predicted	58.4 ± 25.9 (2.3 ± 0.8)	//	//
FEV1% predicted	64 ± 22 (1.8 ± 0.6)	//	//
FEV1/FVC	78.3 ± 7.8	//	//
TLC % predicted	70.2 ± 17.2 (4.5 ± 1.2)	//	//
DLCO % predicted	41.4 ± 15.5	//	//
KCO % predicted	71.3 ± 16.6	//	//

Table 1.
Patient demographic characteristics, smoking status, and functional parameters of the study population.

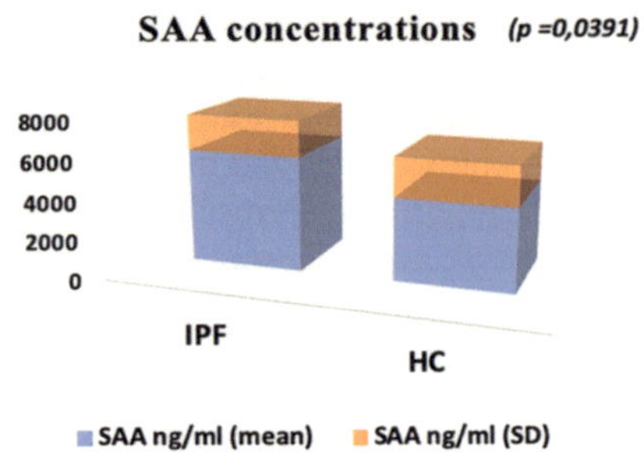

Figure 1.
*Comparison of SAA concentrations between patients with IPF (5890 ± 1852 ng/ml) and healthy controls (4262 ± 2023 ng/ml). IPF, idiopathic pulmonary fibrosis; SAA, serum amyloid A. *p = 0,0391.*

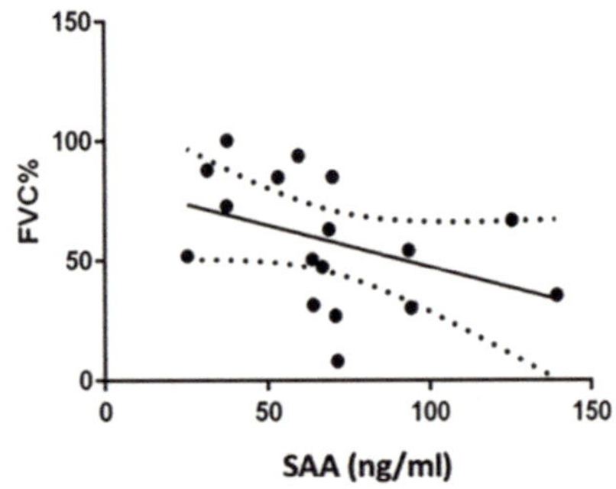

Figure 2.
Correlation between the SAA level and percent FVC in patients with IPF (r = −0,5229; p = 0,015). FVC, forced vital capacity; SAA, serum amyloid A.

IPF patients with a serum SAA concentration above the 75th percentile had worse survival (**Figure 3**).

In our 2019 study, we first presented in the literature the potential profibrotic role of the protein SAA, which has traditionally been known only as an acute-phase protein. As inflammation plays a marginal role in IPF, it is interesting to investigate how SAA might contribute to pulmonary fibrosis. What is known from the literature is that hypoxia (as in the case of OSAS) induces the release of several mediators,

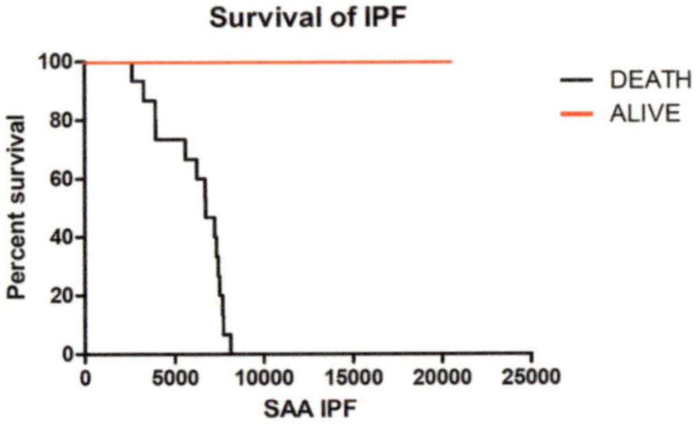

Figure 3.
Kaplan-Meier distribution of survival in patients with idiopathic pulmonary fibrosis and serum amyloid A levels above or below the 75th percentile (p = 0,0018).

including TGF-β, leading to the activation of metalloproteinases (MMP-5, MMP-7, and MMP-1), which in turn activate fibroblasts-myofibroblasts and promote extracellular matrix deposition [3, 14, 20, 22, 45, 46]. The statistically significant and inverse correlation with the percentage of FVC is particularly interesting, as it suggests that SAA could be a prognostic marker of IPF. Indeed, the Kaplan–Meier curve showed that IPF patients with higher serum SAA levels have reduced survival. Thus, SAA might be considered a serum marker for IPF to monitor over time in order to identify stable patients or those with functional progression, who should be closely followed.

Once released into circulation, SAA binds to HDL3, forming a circulating complex with a high affinity for macrophages. The reduction in circulating HDL levels increases the cardiovascular risk in IPF patients (ischemic heart disease, pulmonary hypertension), which are common comorbidities in this patient population [47–49].

To strengthen our hypothesis, we further expanded the study population by measuring the serum concentration of SAA in other fibrosing interstitial lung diseases, including those secondary to connective tissue diseases (data currently under statistical analysis for upcoming publication). Furthermore, to exclude the bias of the age factor (and the possibility that the serum concentration of SAA may increase with age since IPF patients are older than healthy controls), we are analyzing the SAA in serum samples from healthy individuals of the same age as the IPF patients (data currently under statistical analysis for upcoming publication).

3. Conclusion

Our findings about SAA support the hypothesis of such protein as a potential specific biomarker for IPF that can predict clinical course and prognosis of patients. Monitoring SAA serum levels could be useful to identify patients with rapidly progressive IPF disease phenotype (with functional worsening) in order to direct such patients to antifibrotic therapies and lung transplantation earlier. Moreover, it strengthens the hypothesis about the role of lipid metabolism in the fibrotic process. It appears that SAA plays an important role in regulating the fibrotic process (*via* MMPs) and lipid metabolism in IPF patients. Therefore, SAA could be considered a potential specific biomarker for IPF, as well as a possible therapeutic target.

Conflict of interest

The author declare no conflict of interest.

Author details

Lucia Vietri
University Hospital of Ferrara, Italy

*Address all correspondence to: lucia.vietri89@gmail.com

References

[1] Corte TJ, Ellis R, Renzoni EA, Hansell DM, Nicholson AG, du Bois RM, et al. Use of intravenous cyclophosphamide in known or suspected, advanced non-specific interstitial pneumonia. Sarcoidosis, Vasculitis, and Diffuse Lung Diseases. 2009;**26**:132-138

[2] Patel H, Fellowes R, Coade S, Woo P. Human serum amyloid A has cytokine-like properties. Scandinavian Journal of Immunology. 1998;**48**(4):410-418

[3] Yamada T. Serum amyloid A (SAA): A concise review of biology, assay methods and clinical usefulness. Clinical Chemistry and Laboratory Medicine. 1999;**37**(4):381-388

[4] Westermark GT, Engstrom U, Westermark P. The N-terminal segment of protein AA determines its fibrillogenic property. Biochemical and Biophysical Research Communications. 1992;**182**(1):27-33

[5] Jensen LE, Whitehead AS. Regulation of serum amyloid A protein expression during the acute-phase response. The Biochemical Journal. 1998;**334**(Pt 3):489-503

[6] Dwulet FE, Wallace DK, Benson MD. Amino acid structures of multiple forms of amyloid-related serum protein SAA from a single individual. Biochemistry. 1988;**27**(5):1677-1682

[7] Patel H, Bramall J, Waters H, De Beer MC, Woo P. Expression of recombinant human serum amyloid A in mammalian cells and demonstration of the region necessary for high-density lipoprotein binding and amyloid fibril formation by site-directed mutagenesis. The Biochemical Journal. 1996;**318**(Pt 3):1041-1049

[8] Urieli-Shoval S, Linke RP, Matzner Y. Expression and function of serum amyloid a, a major acute-phase protein, in normal and disease states. Current Opinion in Hematology. 2000;**7**(1):64-69

[9] Kluve-Beckerman B, Yamada T, Hardwick J, Liepnieks JJ, Benson MD. Differential plasma clearance of murine acute-phase serum amyloid A proteins SAA1 and SAA2. The Biochemical Journal. 1997;**322**(Pt 2):663-669

[10] Lavie G, Zucker-Franklin D, Franklin EC. Degradation of serum amyloid A protein by surface-associated enzymes of human blood monocytes. The Journal of Experimental Medicine. 1978;**148**(4):1020-1031

[11] Gollaher CJ, Bausserman LL. Hepatic catabolism of serum amyloid A during an acute phase response and chronic inflammation. Proceedings of the Society for Experimental Biology and Medicine. 1990;**194**(3):245-250

[12] Pallotti F, d'Eril GM. La siero amiloide A: biologia ed applicazioni cliniche. Riv Med Lab - JLM. 2003;**4**(1):53-60

[13] Brandwein SR, Medsger TA Jr, Skinner M, Sipe JD, Rodnan GP, Cohen AS. Serum amyloid a protein concentration in progressive systemic sclerosis (scleroderma). Annals of the Rheumatic Diseases. 1984;**43**(4):586-589

[14] Lakota K, Carns M, Podlusky S, Mrak-Poljsak K, Hinchcliff M, Lee J, et al. Serum amyloid A is a marker for pulmonary involvement in systemic sclerosis. PLoS One. 2015;**10**(1):e0110820

[15] Lis-Swiety A, Widuchowska M, Brzezinska-Wcislo L, Kucharz E. High

acute phase protein levels correlate with pulmonary and skin involvement in patients with diffuse systemic sclerosis. The Journal of International Medical Research. 2018;**46**(4):1634-1639

[16] Vallon R, Freuler F, Desta-Tsedu N, Robeva A, Dawson J, Wenner P, et al. Serum amyloid A (apoSAA) expression is up-regulated in rheumatoid arthritis and induces transcription of matrix metalloproteinases. Journal of Immunology. 2001;**166**(4):2801-2807

[17] O'Hara R, Murphy EP, Whitehead AS, FitzGerald O, Bresnihan B. Local expression of the serum amyloid A and formyl peptide receptor-like 1 genes in synovial tissue is associated with matrix metalloproteinase production in patients with inflammatory arthritis. Arthritis and Rheumatism. 2004;**50**(6):1788-1799

[18] Mullan RH, Bresnihan B. Disease-modifying anti-rheumatic drug therapy and structural damage in early rheumatoid arthritis. Clinical and Experimental Rheumatology. 2003;**21**(5 Suppl 31):S158-S164

[19] Mirza S, Clay RD, Koslow MA, Scanlon PD. COPD guidelines: A review of the 2018 GOLD report. Mayo Clinic Proceedings. 2018;**93**(10):1488-1502

[20] Bozinovski S, Hutchinson A, Thompson M, Macgregor L, Black J, Giannakis E, et al. Serum amyloid a is a biomarker of acute exacerbations of chronic obstructive pulmonary disease. American Journal of Respiratory and Critical Care Medicine. 2008;**177**(3):269-278

[21] Bozinovski S, Uddin M, Vlahos R, Thompson M, McQualter JL, Merritt AS, et al. Serum amyloid A opposes lipoxin A(4) to mediate glucocorticoid refractory lung inflammation in chronic obstructive pulmonary disease. Proceedings of the National Academy of Sciences of the United States of America. 2012;**109**(3):935-940

[22] Svatikova A, Wolk R, Shamsuzzaman AS, Kara T, Olson EJ, Somers VK. Serum amyloid A in obstructive sleep apnea. Circulation. 2003;**108**(12):1451-1454

[23] Strohl KP, Brown DB, Collop N, George C, Grunstein R, Han F, et al. An official American Thoracic Society clinical practice guideline: Sleep apnea, sleepiness, and driving risk in noncommercial drivers. An update of a 1994 statement. American Journal of Respiratory and Critical Care Medicine. 2013;**187**(11):1259-1266

[24] Chen SS, Chen FP, Chen XJ. Clinical implications of serum amyloid A level in patients with obstructive sleep apnea. Journal of Southern Medical University. 2009;**29**(8):1599-1601

[25] Bargagli E, Magi B, Olivieri C, Bianchi N, Landi C, Rottoli P. Analysis of serum amyloid A in sarcoidosis patients. Respiratory Medicine. 2011;**105**(5):775-780

[26] Miyoshi S, Hamada H, Kadowaki T, Hamaguchi N, Ito R, Irifune K, et al. Comparative evaluation of serum markers in pulmonary sarcoidosis. Chest. 2010;**137**(6):1391-1397

[27] Chen ES, Song Z, Willett MH, Heine S, Yung RC, Liu MC, et al. Serum amyloid A regulates granulomatous inflammation in sarcoidosis through toll-like receptor-2. American Journal of Respiratory and Critical Care Medicine. 2010;**181**(4):360-373

[28] Chen ES, Moller DR. Etiologies of sarcoidosis. Clinical Reviews in Allergy and Immunology. 2015;**49**(1):6-18

[29] Salazar A, Pinto X, Mana J. Serum amyloid A and high-density

lipoprotein cholesterol: Serum markers of inflammation in sarcoidosis and other systemic disorders. European Journal of Clinical Investigation. 2001;**31**(12):1070-1077

[30] Landi C, Carleo A, Cillis G, Rottoli P. Sarcoidosis: Proteomics and new perspectives for improving personalized medicine. Expert Review of Proteomics. 2018;**15**(10):829-835

[31] Hekking PP, Bel EH. Developing and emerging clinical asthma phenotypes. The Journal of Allergy and Clinical Immunology. In Practice. 2014;**2**(6):671-680

[32] He R, Shepard LW, Chen J, Pan ZK, Ye RD. Serum amyloid A is an endogenous ligand that differentially induces IL-12 and IL-23. Journal of Immunology. 2006;**177**(6):4072-4079

[33] Cheng N, He R, Tian J, Ye PP, Ye RD. Cutting edge: TLR2 is a functional receptor for acute-phase serum amyloid A. Journal of Immunology. 2008;**181**(1):22-26

[34] Ather JL, Ckless K, Martin R, Foley KL, Suratt BT, Boyson JE, et al. Serum amyloid A activates the NLRP3 inflammasome and promotes Th17 allergic asthma in mice. Journal of Immunology. 2011;**187**(1):64-73

[35] Zhang XY, Zhang G, Jiang Y, Liu D, Li MZ, Zhong Q, et al. The prognostic value of serum C-reactive protein-bound serum amyloid A in early-stage lung cancer. Chinese Journal of Cancer. 2015;**34**(8):335-349

[36] Sung HJ, Ahn JM, Yoon YH, Rhim TY, Park CS, Park JY, et al. Identification and validation of SAA as a potential lung cancer biomarker and its involvement in metastatic pathogenesis of lung cancer. Journal of Proteome Research. 2011;**10**(3):1383-1395

[37] Lin HY, Tan GQ, Liu Y, Lin SQ. The prognostic value of serum amyloid A in solid tumors: A meta-analysis. Cancer Cell International. 2019;**19**:62

[38] Zhou J, Sheng J, Fan Y, Zhu X, Tao Q, He Y, et al. Association between serum amyloid A levels and cancers: A systematic review and meta-analysis. Postgraduate Medical Journal. 2018;**94**(1115):499-507

[39] Malle E, Sodin-Semrl S, Kovacevic A. Serum amyloid A: An acute-phase protein involved in tumour pathogenesis. Cellular and Molecular Life Sciences. 2009;**66**(1):9-26

[40] Cho WC, Yip TT, Cheng WW, Au JS. Serum amyloid A is elevated in the serum of lung cancer patients with poor prognosis. British Journal of Cancer. 2010;**102**(12):1731-1735

[41] Zhang Y, Zhang J, Sheng H, Li H, Wang R. Acute phase reactant serum amyloid A in inflammation and other diseases. Advances in Clinical Chemistry. 2019;**90**:25-80

[42] Jana AK, Greenwood AB, Hansmann UHE. Presence of a SARS-COV-2 Protein Enhances Amyloid Formation of Serum Amyloid A. The Journal of Physical Chemistry B. 2021;**125**(32):9155-9167

[43] Zhang D, Huang WJ, Lan MQ, Gan FR, et al. Association between serum amyloid A levels and predicting disease severity in COVID-19 patients: A systematic review and meta-analysis. European Review for Medical and Pharmacological Sciences. 2021;**25**:4627-4638

[44] Raghu G, Remy-Jardin M, Myers JL, Richeldi L, Ryerson CJ, Lederer DJ, et al. Diagnosis of idiopathic pulmonary fibrosis. An official ATS/ERS/JRS/ALAT

clinical practice guideline. Critical Care Medicine. 2018;**198**:e44-e68

[45] Uhlar CM, Whitehead AS. Serum amyloid A, the major vertebrate acute-phase reactant. European Journal of Biochemistry. 1999;**265**:501-523

[46] Pan Y, Fu H, Kong Q, Xiao Y, Shou Q, Chen H, et al. Prevention of pulmonary fibrosis with salvianolic acid a by inducing fibroblast cell cycle arrest and promoting apoptosis. Journal of Ethnopharmacology. 2014;**155**:1589-1596

[47] Benditt EP, Eriksen N. Amyloid protein SAA is associated with high density lipoprotein from human serum. Proceedings of the National Academy of Sciences of the United States of America. 1977;**74**:4025-4028

[48] Salazar A, Mana J, Fiol C, Hurtado I, Argimon JM, Pujol R, et al. Influence of serum amyloid A on the decrease of high density lipoprotein-cholesterol in active sarcoidosis. Atherosclerosis. 2000;**152**:497-502

[49] Dalleywater W, Powell HA, Hubbard RB, Navaratnam V. Risk factors for cardiovascular disease in people with idiopathic pulmonary fibrosis: A population-based study. Chest. 2015;**147**:150-156